Preface

KW-054-388

This book was written for three reasons. First, so that families and caregivers might gain as much information as possible and proceed with their duties in a responsible and loving manner. Secondly, to present my experiences and views in order to further the debate and hopefully make dementia care a better place. The third reason I wrote this book was to show my daughters, Kate and Zoe, what one can do when they put their mind to it.

Wa_____

Practical Dementia For Families and Caregivers

Doug Wornell MD

chipmunkapublishing
the mental health publisher

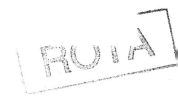

Published by
Chipmunkapublishing
PO Box 6872
Brentwood
Essex CM13 1ZT
United Kingdom

http://www.chipmunkapublishing.com

Chipmunkapublishing gratefully acknowledge the support of Arts Council England.

Author Biography

Douglas Wornell, MD is a geriatric psychiatrist with a large practice in the Seattle-Tacoma area of Washington State, USA. He was born in 1955 in Tacoma and has lived throughout the United States. Dr. Wornell got his bachelor's degree in chemistry at the University of Puget Sound and his medical degree at the University of Miami. He did his internship in general surgery at the Albert Einstein College of Medicine and his residency in psychiatry at St. Luke's Roosevelt Hospital Center in New York City.

Dr. Wornell lived in New York City for 13 years, eventually becoming the Director of Psychiatric Emergency Services for St. Luke's Roosevelt Hospital Center and Assistant Clinical Professor of Psychiatry at Columbia University College of Physicians and Surgeons.

He is now back home in Washington State and is the Medical Director of the Behavioral Wellness Center at Auburn Regional Medical Center. He has participated in the treatment of over twenty thousand dementia patients in the past ten years. Additionally he is the Medical Director of Wornell Psychiatry and Associates, a geriatric and neurological psychiatry consultative service covering over 2000 long term care patients. He has given over 200 presentations on geriatric psychiatry.

Doug Wornell MD

Disclaimer

This book should at no time be considered a substitute for actual care provided by a qualified clinician and is only intended as a resource. I assume no responsibility for treatment decisions or outcomes.

Doug Wornell MD

Forward

The Wandering Explorers

Dementia is a term used to denote deterioration of the brain. The disease process is generally slow and progressive but may vary. While many consider the classic dementia to be Alzheimer's disease, there are many disorders that fall into the broad classification of dementia. The impact of dementia on both the patient and the family is enormous and devastating. This is true not only because of the loss of brain function but also because of the slow and agonizing nature of the disease process itself.

As we age many aspects of our body begin to deteriorate. It is not a surprise therefore that a deteriorative illness such as dementia would most commonly occur in the elderly. It is interesting however that this common aspect of aging is so rarely seen as normal, particularly considering that one sees an uncanny reversal of the developmental milestones seen in youth - infants change into toddlers and then into adolescents in much the same but opposite way that dementia progresses. It is as though the demented brain is falling apart just as it was glued together. One by one, each life experience becomes erased from short-term memory leaving the patient more and more dependent upon the past. Eventually there are no more memories to erase. And then the person we once knew seems gone.

How perfect then for the pharmaceutical industry and research centers to have an illness that will ultimately occur in all of us - if we live long enough. Is it an accident that the dreaded Alzheimer's disease and senile dementia are virtually synonymous terms? If you look at the average age of patients in drug studies for Alzheimer's medications one finds no shortage of very old people represented yet if you compare a

50 year old with this disease and a 90 year old with "Alzheimer's Disease" it appears to be two completely different circumstances. Of course a 50 year old with dementia is clearly abnormal and deserves all the notoriety and research available but, are we being somewhat misguided into being overly concerned about a disease state when we should be more focused upon healthy aging? The somewhat preventable small blood vessel disease component, commonly known as hardening of the arteries and so prevalent in the aging brain, has been left out of the Alzheimer's equation. Yet we sit and watch Erectile Dysfunction commercials on television on a daily basis that clearly show the relationship of small vessel disease from hypertension or diabetes to ED. It would seem we have all wandered and explored ourselves into strange territory. Perhaps the idea of an incurable disease of the penis is just too unacceptable.

Regardless, we are left to ask the question, what must it be like to possess only limited cognitive skills and distant memories of childhood? It's hard to say. Some with dementia seem quite pleasant while others live in misery. This actually doesn't sound too much different than the general population and reminds us that the psychology of dementia is highly influenced by the pre-dementia psychological nature of the patient. But to be sure, the frequency of psychiatric symptoms such as anxiety, depression and psychosis are much more common in the demented population than the general population.

Again I return to the parallel of dementia to developing children. They too seem to exhibit a higher than usual amount of psychiatric symptoms although we don't usually think of it that way. We see it as normal that infants are impulsive, talk to themselves, and are tearful at least three to four times a day. Of course it is normal but what about dementia? Is there a baseline behavioral description that could be considered "normal" for dementia? This question is important because of the longevity of the illness. The process is slow and painful. It can tear people up. Wouldn't it be easier to metabolize some of the emotion involved by accepting the patient at any given point in time for who and where they are, just as we would a child?

I have heard countless family members refer to their demented father or wife as someone who is not the same person they once were. I would argue otherwise. Would you say that your 14 year old was not the same person when they were an infant? Disease or not, dementia is a condition that needs to be contended with as there is a general process of brain deterioration that occurs in all of us as we age. Sooner or later we are less able to react, concentrate and remember as clearly as in years past. We may lose our driving privileges. We are offered help in the home or suggestions to sell the home and move to assisted living. We need reminders. The fact is that one third of all people over the age of 85 have dementia. Ninety percent of all those over age 100 are demented. Are they gone? Are they not the same people? If not, why don't we be honest with ourselves and eliminate them. It would save billions and limit grief. The reason is simple. We know they are the same people. It is, however difficult to witness the drama of deterioration. We defend ourselves by seeing them as someone else.

Wandering explorers is a term I use those with moderate to severe dementia. It suggests a cognitive limitation and yet notes a purpose in behavior and activity. As with children, we have a responsibility to see that these explorers are as content and healthy as possible. Dementia care requires no less sensitivity or sophistication of care than that in the management of children.

After acceptance, we shall find other important ways to manage patients with dementia. Some of these are minimizing medication, maximizing appropriate social stimulation, and continuously being prepared for change.

Older people have multiple medical problems and are often on several medications. They also have limited tolerance to medications and most will sooner or later require some psychiatric medication. As we shall see, one way of minimizing medication is through ample amounts of social stimulation and structure. And change is perhaps the most important aspect of dementia to become accustomed to. Nothing is ever certain with dementia. It is in constant evolution. Simple events like a room change or a urinary tract infection may cause chaos.

In this book we will embark on an exploration of our own. We shall look deeper into issues of acceptance, psychology and the dynamics of dementia. We shall separate the realities from the myths and answer some basic questions like how dementia starts and how those with it die. We'll talk about family reactions and common dilemmas such as how the healthy spouse deals with guilt and fears of being alone. Finally, we'll take a look at some practical matters such as psychiatric medication, planning and placement considerations.

Chapter 1

What is dementia?

Dementia is one of several categories of neurological disorders that make up a general classification known as Organic Brain Syndromes or Organic Mental Syndromes (OBS or OMS). These different categories of organic brain syndromes are often interrelated making it necessary to mention the others too. Delirium, for example, is commonplace in demented patients. We shall address this entity throughout the book and pay particular attention to it in another chapter. Mental retardation and traumatic brain injury are also defined as organic brain disorders. They too have a relationship with dementia and shall be mentioned throughout as they are often found to either promote the development of dementia or are misidentified as such.

The word "organic" is actually an old term born out of an era when causes of psychiatric problems were less well understood. Thus the more neurologic disorders with palpable or measurable changes in the brain such as dementia, delirium, brain trauma and mental retardation were labeled as "organic" illnesses. The mental illnesses such as schizophrenia, bipolar illness and depression were labeled as "functional".

Interestingly, schizophrenia, a classic "functional" or psychiatric illness was originally named dementia praecox. This reflects an even earlier period when there were no psychiatrists. Neurologists, such as Sigmund Freud, were effectively the medical experts in all mental conditions. Many with such disorders were not only seen as demented but also given other diagnoses that are now words of diminution such as imbeciles, idiots and morons. I would refer disbelievers to any early nineteen hundreds medical text.

In the end, dementia is now considered to be an organic or neurological illness that very commonly has an associated psychiatric component such as depression, anxiety or psychosis.

If we accept the notion of organic brain disease as involving measurable changes in the brain then dementia is well placed in this category. Senile dementia, a term pretty much used synonymously with Alzheimer's disease (AD), involves a very clear shrinkage of the brain called atrophy. In vascular dementia there are multiple small (or large) areas of strokes also known as infarcts. Lewy Body dementia involves small protein bodies in the brain cells known as Lewy Bodies. The list goes on and on with each type of dementia having distinct and recognizable brain tissue defects where, on a more microscopic level brain cells and\or their connections are dying.

While many particular brain changes have been described, the root cause of most cases of dementia remains mysterious. For example, there is no known cause for the degenerative process that unfolds in Alzheimer's disease. It seems obvious to me that the older the population we are talking about is, the more likely the "the disease" is confused or at least complicated by normal aging issues. And these aging changes are complex as well.

There are two processes that seem to stand out as being linked with brain aging. One is oxidation and the formation of unstable molecules known as free radicals. It may be helpful to realize that another well-known form of oxidation is rust. In response to this there has been a great deal of emphasis upon nutritional changes in our diets containing proper amounts of exercise, vitamins, omega 3 fatty acids and other substances such as resveratrol in red wine, blackberries and blue berries. The other process that seems to occur in most aging organs is the development of atherosclerosis or fatty plaques that ultimately lead to strokes or areas of dead tissue beyond a blockage. As stated, this is commonly known as hardening of the arteries and is well known to be associated with high blood pressure, diabetes and high cholesterol. Other illnesses such as heart attack and stroke have also been linked with atherosclerosis thus sounding the alarm for dietary changes with less red meat, better control of blood pressure and diabetes and more exercise with less cigarette smoking.

In its pure form, vascular or stroke dementia therefore seems to be better understood if one considers the risk factors that are associated with the fatty plaques of arteriosclerosis and subsequent stroke formation. Some dementia is related to metabolism such as Wilson's disease with copper metabolism while others are related to nutrition like vitamin B12 deficiency. Other dementia such as Huntington's disease (Woody Guthrie's misfortune) is purely genetic while others have clear environmental causes such as that associated with chronic alcohol use. Dementia can be caused by an infectious virus like in HIV dementia, a later stage of the bacterial illness syphilis (Al Capone's fatal illness) or the human variant of mad cow disease known as Cruetzfeltd-Jacob disease. The infectious agent in this disease is called a prion.

In all cases brain cells or their connections are destroyed. The damage typically occurs over time and is initially non-lethal. Indeed, it is this slow and initially non-fatal loss of the mental function that gives these diseases their hallmarks – years of complex and expensive medical care, continuous family struggles around grief and acceptance, and long term placement issues.

By far the major risk factor for the development of dementia is age. Eighty percent of all dementia occurring in the world is in patients sixty and older. Most of these are Alzheimer's disease, vascular dementia or Lewy Body dementia. Great effort is made amongst clinicians and scientists to separate these three illnesses into individual syndromes with identifiable criteria. It is the nature of science and medicine to do so and serves a purpose of further understanding and ultimately treating these maladies. Unfortunately it serves less purpose from a current practical point of view. Treatments are similar although important differences do exist and combination disease is common. For example up to 50% of Alzheimer cases have vascular changes discovered on autopsy.

In the end it is Alzheimer's disease that has gained the most notoriety in the US. Most academic centers agree that around 60% of all cases of dementia in the US are caused by this degenerative illness. The mere fact that Alzheimer's is synonymous with senile dementia speaks to its first position in the hierarchy of dementias as age is so closely associated dementia is general. But if hardening of the arteries is so closely linked to age as well and strokes are known to be associated with hardening of the arteries then why not more press about stroke or vascular dementia?

Like dementia, diseases of fatty plaques formation or atherosclerosis are more common in the elderly. Heart attacks (MI - Myocardial infarctions) and strokes (CVA – cerebro-vascular accidents) are closely associated with arteriosclerosis. Heart attacks kill heart muscle and are a major contributor to a weakening of the heart as a pump and thus congestive heart failure. Isn't this in effect a sort of senile dementia of the heart? Again, why then isn't vascular dementia more synonymous with senile dementia of the brain. When you think about it, isn't it a little strange that a degenerative illness of no known cause is the major cause of deterioration of the most highly vascularized organ in our body when vascular changes are staring us in the face.

Let's argue the point further. There are vascular or blood vessel risks that are actually associated with Alzheimer's dementia such as high homocysteine levels. Even the major genetic link to Alzheimer's disease, having the AOPO E4 protein genotype, is actually used by cardiologists to screen for atherosclerotic disease of the heart. Our experience is that most patients with "senile" dementia who are more than eighty years have more than one risk factor for vascular dementia such as diabetes or high blood pressure.

Without question, Alzheimer's disease does exist and is a major contributor to the dementia we see in the world. It seems clear however, that many cases of blood vessel related dementia are misdiagnosed as Alzheimer's disease. It is important because Alzheimer's disease is not felt to be preventable whereas much of vascular disease related maladies are. Rather than having the world waiting around for CNN to report a cure for Alzheimer's disease that is unlikely to happen soon, more efforts could be placed on medical and nutritional care with healthy blood vessels in mind as it relates not just to heart attacks and strokes but also dementia. Unfortunately, microscopic blood vessel disease or small stroke disease is not a commonly accepted criterion for stroke dementia. Rather, there must be evidence of an actual larger stroke to be labeled as vascular dementia.

So, for better or worse, it is Alzheimer's disease that has caught the eye of the public, the pharmaceutical industry, research, and the long-term care industry. The baby boomers are coming of age now and the dementia industry is gearing up to prepare for the expected rise in the need for Alzheimer care. It is estimated that the 3 million in the US now with the disease will grow to 15 million by 2050. New medications for Alzheimer's have come out in the past ten years and that is only the beginning. The acceptance of these medications as means to delay symptom progression of dementia is increasing. There is more and more talk in research circles about managing the risk factors for atherosclerosis as it relates to dementia.

Soon long term and dementia care facilities will become more common. Already more and more assisted living facilities and skilled nursing facilities are specializing in dementia care. Despite most dementia patients being cared for by families at home there are many who cannot be. This is partly because of behavioral reasons but also that dementia patients are older and can have complex medical issues. Such facilities can not only provide medical or behavioral care but also give the social stimulation and structure that is so therapeutically important in the treatment of dementia.

Chapter 2

Alzheimer's disease

As previously stated, Alzheimer's disease (AD) and senile dementia are synonymous terms. We have discussed how this may be an unfortunate association as there is evidence that the process most closely associated with senility is atherosclerosis. Microvascular changes (damage caused by microscopic strokes) rather than a degenerative process of unknown cause like AD might better be named senile dementia if it weren't for the strict criteria of making the diagnosis of vascular dementia whereby an actual larger stroke must have occurred. In any event, like vascular dementia, the primary risk for AD is age. There are also genetic links in AD but these appear to be involving more than one gene as compared with a disease like Huntington's where a single gene has been proven to transmit the illness. There is no known environmental cause of AD nor is there a parenting style that will produce a child who will later develop senile dementia.

AD has been traditionally thought to be a disease of the cortex or gray matter of the brain. It is therefore also known to be a "cortical" dementia. The cortex is where the actual brain cells or neurons are. The white matter or subcortical area is beneath the gray matter and is filled with connection fibers between the brain cells. In AD there is a particular loss of function in an area called the hippocampus, a primary short term memory center in the brain. The cholinergic system mediated by a chemical called Acetylcholine (ACH) is also destroyed. ACH is one of many neurotransmitters that provide for transmission of messages between nerve cells. ACH is found through the body but plays a vital role in memory and other cognitive functions.

The loss of brain cells and their function is progressive in AD. The gross result is shrinkage of the mass of the brain. This can readily be seen with imaging studies and is called atrophy. While this is to some degree a normal finding in the elderly, generalized atrophy of the brain is always suggestive of AD particularly in a younger patient.

The cause of pure AD is unknown. Until very recently a good explanation of the major mechanism of the disease went something like this: for some reason dormant cells called glia, a kind of connective tissue in the brain, come to life and secrete a plaque called beta amyloid that is toxic to the brain's functional cells or neurons. An inflammatory process ensues around the neuron and kills it.

More recently the exact role of this plaque formation has come into question particularly after some animal studies demonstrated that reversal of the plaque formation does not reverse the disease. It is not thought to be a much more complex puzzle that may involve more of the connection fibers between the cells rather than the actual neurons themselves.

Still, a microscopic autopsy finding that is typical of AD is an abundance of "senile plaques" which is the beta amyloid protein that has been secreted. Another finding is called neurofibrillary tangles. These tangles are the twisted remnants of the tubular transport system between the cells that becomes disrupted as well.

Other than looking at the brain under the microscope there is not a single diagnostic test that is indicative of AD. Since we are not doing brain biopsies on each patient suspected of having AD, the diagnosis is made through a careful inventory of the history, examination, and supportive information from a brain scan. Delirium, or acute medical confusion, must always be ruled out. Chronic mental illness is excluded. New onset mental illness such as anxiety or depression can often masquerade as dementia. Unfortunately these symptoms may well be a part of the dementia syndrome itself making for a complicated diagnostic dilemma. In fact, the depression for example, may need to be addressed before the diagnosis can be made. In the end however the short term memory loss of AD will give it away. This memory loss is more severe and persistent than that found in depression and anxiety.

There are a few illnesses known as "reversible dementias" that are commonly tested for but the results are usually negative. We shall discuss these later. Finally, other types of dementia are considered - in particular, vascular and Lewy body dementia. In a relatively young patient of sixty years who has progressive memory loss with little to support a medical cause, vascular dementia or Lewy body disease (discussed later), there is little else it could be but Alzheimer's disease or some much less common dementia.

In general, AD will involve a progressive loss of short term memory in a person beyond fifty years of age that significantly interferes with the activities of daily living (ADLs). A patient jokingly worried about his memory loss probably does not have this dementia. Mild memory loss associated with age is normal. Memory loss associated with AD is frightening and devastating.

It is ironic that this frightening aspect of the memory loss in AD often makes the diagnosis difficult to make. Afflicted persons will rarely seek help for it but rather try to hide it. This will eventually become unintentional. As the memory loss progresses the patient has less and less awareness of the problem. Family members and friends are frequently aware early on but nothing is said due to the sensitive subject and the chance of a confrontation met with resistance. Additionally, few are aware of the importance of early detection. It will often require the emergence of secondary psychiatric symptoms or further disorganization before someone finally does something.

Psychiatric symptoms may be a direct result of attempts to navigate the cognitive decline in what is viewed as an increasingly hostile world. They include depression, anxiety, obsessions, paranoia, and hostile defensiveness.

The spouse will often be the object of misguided hostility as the emotionally charged relationship becomes contorted and twisted in the mind of the one stricken with the dementing illness.

Let's look at an example. Grandma becomes obsessed with taking a drive each day up the highway towards the mountain. The granddaughter, with whom she lives, complies and takes her. After a week of daily drives grandma seems more depressed as she begins to ask questions about where the old house was. Her eating decreases and her sleep is disturbed. The granddaughter isn't sure where the old house was but promises to call her mother and ask. This creates hopelessness in grandma and anxiety begins during the trip. Back at home granddaughter calms her with a glass of wine. Granddaughter questions grandma about the drives and need to see the old house. Grandma gets defensive and begins to argue with her feeling it's none her business. They begin to quarrel.

What is happening? Grandma is losing her short-term memory. In an attempt to keep herself oriented and lower the level of anxiety, her mind defensively seeks a long-term memory to familiarize herself. When this fails to square with reality she gets depressed at first and then desperate. No doubt it is depressing to sense that your memory is failing. Note how the defensiveness heightens when the granddaughter begins to ask questions. This denial and defensiveness is typical of early AD. Obviously it can make the diagnosis and treatment difficult. Only the rare patient walks through the door looking for treatment of such symptoms as they might have with a headache.

Obviously, this example illustrates a very important clinical aspect of AD. Although initially an illness of memory failure, the presentation may well be secondary symptoms like depression, anxiety or paranoia. The family may only later report the memory loss. On many occasions it requires a health professional to complete a mental status examine before the memory impairment is uncovered. This will be discussed further in a later chapter.

Unfortunately, this is only the beginning. AD is a progressive illness that will ultimately do just that - progress. Let's look at the DSM IV criteria for making the diagnosis of AD. The DSM IV (Diagnostic and Statistical Manual of Mental Disorders) is the American Psychiatric Association's standard for mental health diagnoses. It is commonly used as a standard for making the diagnosis of AD.

Dementia of Alzheimer's Type   294.1 (DSM IV diagnosis code)

> A. The development of multiple cognitive deficits manifested by both
>
> 1) Memory impairment (impaired ability to learn new information or to recall previously learned information)
> 2)   One (or more) of the following cognitive disturbances:
>
> > a)   Aphasia (language disturbance)
> > b)   Apraxia (impaired ability to carry out motor activities despite intact motor function)
> > c)   Agnosia (failure to recognize or identify objects despite intact sensory function)

    d) Disturbance in executive functioning (i.e., planning, organizing, sequencing, abstracting)

B. The cognitive deficits in Criteria A1 and A2 each cause significant impairment of social or occupational functioning and represent a significant decline from a previous level of functioning.

C. The course is characterized by gradual onset and continuing cognitive decline.

D. The cognitive deficits in Criteria A1 and A2 are not due to any of the following:

    1) Other central nervous system conditions that cause progressive deficits in memory and cognition (e.g., cerebrovascular disease, Parkinson's disease, Huntington's disease, subdural hematoma, normal-pressure hydrocephalus, brain tumor)

    2) Systemic conditions that are known to cause dementia (e.g., hypothyroidism, vitamin B12 deficiency or folic acid deficiency, niacin deficiency, hypercalcemia, neurosyphilis, HIV infection)

    3) Substance-induced conditions

E. The deficits do not occur exclusively during the course of delirium.

F. The disturbance is not better accounted for by another Axis I disorder (e.g., Major Depressive Disorder, Schizophrenia)

Thus far we have discussed psychiatric symptoms in addition to the memory loss. As you can see these symptoms such as depression or anxiety are not parts of the diagnosis and only listed late in the DSM IV as something to rule out before you can make the diagnosis of AD. In practice however, they are very commonly associated with AD. Not only are they often the initial sign that something is wrong but may become more frequent throughout the course of the disease.

Sooner or later, the short-term memory deteriorates further and other brain functions become involved. Dementia has usually been diagnosed by the time that spatial orientation, recognition, concentration, calculation and other primary skills decline. This decline will lead to more drastic unconscious defensive measures to deal with a very fragmented world. We are, at this point, entering the realm of possible psychotic thinking. Psychosis is a distortion of reality. It may involve a hallucination (distortion of perception), a delusion (distortion of thought content), or a looseness of association (distortion of thought process). Dementia may involve one or all of these. The grandmother previously described patient may soon be hearing her mother's voice, having paranoid delusions of plots by family members and thoughts so loose and tangential that they are hard for both patient and family to follow.

Ultimately, there is physical decline. Increase disorganized wandering and weakness may lead to a fall. Disorganized eating may lead to aspiration (inhaling food) and then pneumonia. Disorganized hygiene may lead to a urinary infection or sores. Compliance with medication declines and other medical problems become unstable. AD does not directly kill its victims as much as provide for enough of a physical decline to perish of other causes.

AD is a slow and progressive illness with high financial and emotion cost to both patients and families. On average, the disease may last five to ten years from start to finish. There appears to be some preference of AD for women however women live longer and may be more likely to become demented for this reason. In fact, we all seem to be at a higher risk for AD as we are all living longer. Age remains the primary risk for AD. As previously stated, it is currently estimated that one third of those eighty five have AD. Studies have been done on one hundred year olds and have found that some ninety percent have dementia. We have discussed that, based upon such statistics, that one might wonder if dementia in the elderly that may be diagnosed as AD may be a natural part of getting older. What is very clear is that when a 50 or 60 year old, with few or no cardiovascular risk factors gets AD, it is an absolute nightmare.

Whichever it is, the percentage of the total population that is elderly is rising. The baby boomers are now on the cusp of disease. It is estimated that the 4 to 5 million cases of dementia we see now in the US shall rise to 15 to 20 million by 2050. In recent years there has been developed a diagnosis called MCI or minimal cognitive impairment. This is a diagnosis developed by neurologists to help identify AD in its earliest stages. These are cases of more severe memory loss than that usual found with aging but without the loss of activities of daily living social functioning. Research has shown that many such cases will develop into AD. It is important to recognize AD as early as possible because the current medications that directly treat AD work best if started early. We shall discuss them in detail later.

There is a small group of AD cases that are called "familial". In such instances families pass the disease from generation to generation. These cases of familial AD tend to have an earlier onset and be a more aggressive form of the illness. But they represent only ten percent of the cases of AD and are understood to be the result of mutant genes being past on. There are another sixty percent of cases of AD known as "sporadic" that carry a particular gene type that codes for a protein called APO-E. APO-E comes in different genotypes labeled APO-E 1, 2, 3 or 4. We get one APO-E gene from each parent. We might therefore have a combination of one APO-E2 and one APO-E3. It turns out that if you have one APO-E4 you'll have about 4 times the risk of having AD. If you have two APO-E4s you'll have about 11 times the chance of developing AD. And again, the vascular dementia issue enters the picture. It turns out that APO-E4 is also associated with cardiovascular disease and atherosclerosis. It remains unclear how many of the cases diagnosed as AD in the genetic studies for AD and APO-E4 actually had a vascular component. While some cardiology centers are using APO-E gene testing to screen for potential heart disease it is not currently being used to screen for AD.

Chapter 3

Vascular dementia

Vascular or stroke related dementia is generally considered to be the second or third most common form of dementia in the United States. Most academic centers in the U.S. say it accounts for about 15 to 20% of our dementia. This is not the case in other parts of the world where, in Japan for example, vascular types of dementia are diagnosed more often than Alzheimer dementia. The word vascular suggests something to do with the blood vessels. An infarction, as in multi-infarct dementia, is an area of tissue damaged by lack of blood supply. A stroke is a form of an infarction. Therefore multi-infarct dementia is caused by multiple strokes.

There are different types of dementia thought to be the result of vascular problems. Differentiating them seems to have to do with the size of the damaged area or stroke. The other has to do with whether the predominant areas of damage are cortical, subcortical or both. Remember that Alzheimer's disease is a cortical dementia. Therefore, memory loss and a decline in cognitive abilities usually predominates the clinical presentation. Psychiatric symptoms in AD may occur early on but are usually a psychological reaction to the cognitive deterioration. In stroke dementia, the direct result of damage to potentially all levels of brain tissue may cause the mood instability itself. This may well me early on. Therefore a stroke or vascular dementia frequently presents as an unstable mood having periods of ups, downs, yelling and distress.

Depression is extremely common in any stroke disease and that includes vascular dementia. In fact mood problems are so closely linked to stroke disease that studies have shown very clear benefits of anti-depressant therapy in such patients relative to survival. A 2003 multi-national study showed a

75% 9 year survival rate in stroke patients treated with antidepressants early on after the stroke compared with a 25% 9 year survival in those who weren't. Let's now look at the DSM IV definition of vascular dementia.

Vascular Dementia   290.4

A. The Development of multiple cognitive deficits manifested by both

1) Memory impairment (impaired ability to learn new information or to recall previously learned information)

2) One (or more) of the following cognitive disturbances:

a) Aphasia (language disturbance)

b) Apraxia (impaired ability to carry out motor activities despite intact motor function)

c) Agnosia (failure to recognize or identify objects despite intact sensory function)

d) Disturbance in executive functioning (i.e., planning, organizing, sequencing, abstracting)

B. The cognitive deficits in A1 and A2 each cause significant impairment in social or occupational functioning and represent a significant decline from a previous level of functioning.

C. Focal neurological signs and symptoms (e.g., exaggeration of deep tendon reflexes, extensor plantar response, pseudo bulbar palsy, gait

> abnormalities, weakness of an extremity) or laboratory evidence indicative of cerebrovascular disease (e.g., multiple infarctions involving the cortex and underlying white matter) that are judged to be etiologically related to the disturbance.
>
> D. The deficits do not occur exclusively during the course of a delirium.

Remember that vascular dementia is a broad term used to describe a dementia caused by blood vessel disease. Note that the primary difference in the DSM IV definition of AD versus vascular dementia is item C. In AD a progressive decline is described. A progressive decline will inevitably occur in vascular dementia as well however the point being made is that the nature of the progression may be different and there may be other neurologic symptoms such as weakness or paralysis associated with it. In vascular dementia the progression of confusion is commonly stepwise in nature with huge advances in the level of confusion literally happening overnight at times. This is because of the nature of vascular events. A stroke, large or small often arrives suddenly and so does the syndrome associated with it. It really depends upon what part of the brain is affected. There may initially be confusion, weakness on one side, or even fall. The family and doctor may also be confused about what is going on. The patient with vascular dementia is often left with a new and lower level of brain functioning after the acute episode clears. This is the wickedness of cerebrovascular or stroke disease.

Note that this cerebrovascular disease is listed under item C in the DSM IV. There is controversy here in the medical community and I have not been hesitant to mention it earlier. While the DSM IV places vascular dementia into one large category there are many researchers and clinicians who do not. Many academic centers do not consider a dementia to be purely of vascular origin unless there is an actual stroke. This is important, as a majority of patients with dementia over 70 years of age have an abnormal vascular finding on their brains scans not considered to be a stroke. This finding is labeled differently by radiologists interpreting the CAT or MRI scan and is almost always left out of the report to families. While families are told there is "no acute" change or disease such as a stroke or bleed or tumor, there is, in the small print of the report very commonly a description of patchy areas felt to be microscopic areas of damaged tissue due to troubled blood vessels. Again, the actual language used may vary but is usually stated as small vessel disease, periventricular white matter disease, or chronic ischemic changes. This exclusion may be one reason that Alzheimer's disease is much more commonly diagnosed than vascular dementia.

While the jury is out as to the exact significance of this small stroke disease, it seems clear to me that the vast majority of patients with dementia have small vessel disease. This is especially true of older patients and those with risk factors for atherosclerosis such as hypertension, diabetes and high cholesterol. Fortunately, there seems to be more and more "buzz" in the literature discussing this issue and at least recognizing combined disease is important. As I have said, the primary importance seems to lay with the fact that most risk factors for development of atherosclerosis are treatable. It is true that genetic predispositions vary but there is really no excuse to be walking around with high blood pressure, high cholesterol or blood sugars out of control.

Another risk for stroke disease we have not touched upon but must is atrial fibrillation (AF). This is a quivering of the top chamber of the heart causing the pooling and potential clotting of blood there. The clots may then break free and travel up the carotid artery lodging somewhere above and certainly causing a stroke. For this reason, most people with AF are on a blood thinner such as Coumadin.

In the end, there is no dispute that stroke disease may lead to dementia. It may be associated with a single large stroke in an area of the brain involved with cognitive functioning or multiple smaller strokes also called lacunar infarcts that may be spread throughout the brain. And we have discussed that the greatest threat of all may be on a microvascular level. In any event, the damaged areas may be more cortical (gray matter) and present with memory deficits or more subcortical (white matter) and present with mood instability and\or an attention deficit. A combination cortical and sub-cortical stroke disease is not uncommon.

Other rarer forms of vascular dementia include Binswanger's disease and CADASIL. The former is a microvascular disease of the brain always associated with high blood pressure. The latter, also known as Cortical Autosomal Dominant Disease and Sub-acute Ischemic Leukencephalopathy, is a genetic vascular dementia passed on from one generation to the next.

So, like Alzheimer's disease, older age is the major risk factor for vascular dementia. Different, however, is the association with fatty plaques or atherosclerotic changes in the blood vessels and the ultimate development of areas of damage that account for the illness. Atherosclerosis is a common process whereby plaques composed of fat and cholesterol adhere to the inner walls of arteries. This process begins early in life and has even been found in autopsied children. As the years go by, the plaques increase. The question becomes, how much? Given that atherosclerotic related disease is the number one killer of people in the US, those of us fortunate enough to have minimal plaque formation will likely live longer lives. Those of us who will develop greater amounts of plaques will likely die earlier from some associated vascular disease such as heart attack, stroke, or dementia. Other associated diseases include congestive heart failure, peripheral vascular disease, chronic kidney insufficiency, and erectile dysfunction. In all cases the particular organ in question becomes inundated with strokes and is rendered dysfunctional. To review, the risks for development of atherosclerosis include genetics, diabetes, high blood pressure, high cholesterol. High fat diets, obesity, lack of exercise and cigarette smoking have also been linked.

This business of atherosclerotic plaques and their development is complex and huge research fodder as you might imagine. This is particularly true given that there is some evidence of reversibility. The mechanism of damage to the tissue seems to be less of a stretch. The plaques, sometimes with a little help from blood clots, block arteries. Everything beyond is left with little or no blood supply and dies. This is not reversible. In the case of coronary artery disease, the number one killer of people in the US, the coronary arteries that supply blood to the heart muscle become partially blocked. With the addition of a spasm or a piece of moving broken off plaque or blood clot called an embolus, there can be a sudden total blockage. As we have seen, the damaged area beyond the block is called an infarction. In this case, because it is heart muscle, it is called a myocardial infarction or MI. Slow and sudden blockages can also occur in arteries that supply the in the lower extremities leading to the need for bypass surgery or amputation. This problem is commonly seen in diabetes, a leading contributor to atherosclerotic disease.

The brain uses more blood pound for pound than any other organ. The carotid arteries are the main arteries from the heart that feed the brain with blood. These arteries too can become blocked over time. Ultimately the blockage can become as great as to directly interfere with blood supply to the brain. In such cases a procedure known as carotid endarterectomy may be required to clean out the inside of these vessels. Not uncommonly, small emboli composed of the fatty plaques break away from the carotids and lodge in various places in the brain. A large piece may cause a large area of the brain to lose blood supply creating a stroke. This is also known as a cerebrovascular accident (CVA). This may cause a variety of neurologic symptoms like paralysis or sensory deficits depending upon where the stroke is.

Less spectacular but perhaps more common, small pieces of plaque break away over time causing much smaller areas of strokes. These may not be symptomatic by themselves but eventually take their toll on the neurons. This is a manner in which vascular dementia develops. Additionally, the walls of the arteries in the brain weaken because of the fatty plaques leading to the possibility of bleeding. Also, uncontrolled high blood pressure will cause microscopic areas of bleeding that in effect behave like small hemorrhagic strokes themselves. The end result is damage to the brain tissue from lack of organized blood supply.

As we have discussed, vascular dementia can be associated with a sudden step like advancement where families might be witness to drastic and permanent mental changes literally overnight. This unfortunate phenomenon occurs when a shower of small emboli break away and lodge upstream deep in the brain tissue killing vast amounts of brain tissue over a wide area all at once. The causes of this sad event can range from the continuous pounding of high blood pressure or a traumatic fall to virtually no known cause other than the possibility of pre-existing plaques.

Because vascular dementia is often associated with stroke many such victims are struggling with a variety of neurologic symptoms. We have seen that these can include paralysis, loss of sensation and aphasia. Aphasia is the inability to speak due to damage at the level of the brain. It is commonly associated with a stroke on the left side of the brain where the speech center most often resides. Such a stroke commonly results in a right-sided paralysis because the nerves cross over. Aphasia may be called expressive when the right words won't come out or receptive when the words of others can't be understood. In some cases a global aphasia is diagnosed. Here, the patient cannot give out or receive information. They are frustrated and often agitated. This situation is a complete clinical nightmare scenario. The patient may or may not be confused, there is no way to tell, and it may be permanent. Even in lesser degrees of aphasia the degree of cognitive impairment can be hard to determine and will always complicate the future of the victim with frustration and difficulties with communication.

Another elusive phenomenon, somewhat specific to cerebrovascular disease, is neurologic crying. In such cases a patient may cry and appear very depressed. On examination however, they may report that they do not feel sad and have no idea why they are crying. Imagine the dilemma of understanding what might be going on with an aphasic patient with such crying. Obviously, managing patients with cerebrovascular disease can be one of the greatest challenges of dementia care.

Chapter 4

Lewy body disease

Lewy bodies are protein bodies found in the brain cells of patients with Parkinson's disease (PD) and a form of dementia called Lewy Body dementia or DLB (Dementia with Lewy Bodies). Some consider PD and DLB to be on a continuum although there are some clear differences in the appearance of the Lewy bodies themselves in the two diseases.

PD is in essence a movement disorder that will often progress to include a dementia in its later stages. DLB begins with a dementia and will often involve a Parkinson like movement disorder its later stages. In a sense the two diseases tend towards a similar final picture each having elements of dementia and the movement disorder. The majority of cases of each disease however, remain distinct throughout its evolution.

DLB is considered to be the second or third most common form of dementia depending upon whether or not one considers vascular dementia more common. DLB appears to have elements of a cortical and subcortical dementia. Memory loss and mood issues are a part of the syndrome however fluctuations in levels of attention are a defining element of DLB. PD dementia is more of a pure subcortical dementia and often appears to be more loaded with mood issues, in particular, depression. In fact, depression is very commonly a part of the presentation of PD in general. Therefore, while many of the clinical aspects of Lewy body disease are similar to those of other dementias, there are some unique characteristics that are useful in making the diagnosis. I have mentioned attention and depression which we shall get into further but probably the most important defining element of these disorders has do with a movement disorder.

PD, also known as Paralysis Agitans, is a common neurological illness caused by a dysfunction in an area of the brain known as the basal ganglia. This part of the brain is responsible for the fine-tuning and coordination of muscle movements throughout the body. Much of the proper function of this area of the brain is dependent upon a chemical known as dopamine. Dopamine is one of many neurotransmitters that relay messages between brain cells. It is very much involved in fine motor control as described above but also with thinking. It is this commonality of dopamine's involvement with both movement and thinking that creates a clinical problem in the treatment of DLB and PD dementia.

In PD one finds a relative blockage of dopamine in the basal ganglia. Probably not coincidentally, in PD there is a congregation of the intracellular protein filled Lewy bodies in this part of the brain. The result is a progressive neurologic disease with some very classic symptoms, in part, caused by the protein dis-regulation and secondary inflammatory response of the Lewy bodies themselves.

A very slow frequency shaking tremor of the extremities is classic. The tremor characteristically is greater on one side than the other and rarely involves the head. A pill rolling movement of the hands and fingers is common. The extremities are rigid. There is a slowness to initiate and end movements. The gait is often described as shuffling and the face can have a "mask" or dis-animated quality to it. As stated above, depression is very common in PD and ultimately, so is dementia.

It should be noted too, that Parkinsonism or Parkinson like symptoms can occur in he elderly without a full blown diagnosis of PD. This feature is common in DLB. This is particularly true when antipsychotic medications are used. Such medications are commonly used in the treatment of all forms of dementia because psychosis common in the condition. As stated earlier, dopamine helps to mediate thinking. Anti-psychotic medication works by blocking dopamine so as to minimize psychotic thoughts. Unfortunately, these medications generally are not specific to the areas of the brain that create thought. Other areas such as the basal ganglia or movement centers are affected by the dopamine blockade too.

As you might imagine then, anti-psychotic medication can actually create a Parkinson-like picture as a side effect. This problem is generally reversible with discontinuation of the medication but clearly a patient who already has low dopamine levels such as those with PD or DLB would be very sensitive to these medications. This makes the treatment of psychosis in those with these two disorders especially problematic. From a diagnostic standpoint, any patient with dementia who is particularly sensitive to an antipsychotic medication and does not have a formal diagnosis of PD should be considered to have DLB.

There is no single test for PD or DLB. They are progressive illnesses that can occur in either sex and in any race. Once again, the major risk factor is age. They each may evolve quickly over one year or slowly over ten or more years. The Lewy bodies do not show up on a brain scan or blood test and can only be identified with actual brain tissue under the microscope. Again, we are not doing brain biopsies to make dementia diagnoses therefore a careful history and physical findings form the major roadmap towards understanding what is going on. In the case of PD dementia, the dementia must occur after PD has already been an established disorder in the patient...usually for years. DLB is more often mis-diagnosed so let's look more closely at that.

DLB can be readily diagnosed using the following criteria for any patient with dementia: 1) Parkinsonism (but not PD) or sensitivity to antipsychotic medication, 2) visual hallucinations, and 3) alterations or fluctuations in awareness or attention. Obviously treating the hallucinations with antipsychotic medication is problematic in DLB patients because of the side effects. We shall soon see that there are some anti-psychotics better tolerated in these patients than others.

The third part of the triad, the attention deficit fluctuations, can be quite dramatic. Families will often describe the patient as being back and forth between total alertness and awareness several times throughout the day. These fluctuations should not be confused with the daily worsening of confusion in the afternoon and evening that is commonly seen in senile and vascular dementia. That phenomenon is called sun downing. We shall discuss it in more detail later.

Consider also that all PD patients are treated with medications for their movement disorder and can get psychotic symptoms as side effects from them - including visual hallucinations. Anti-psychotic medication may be needed in such cases because stopping the PD medication is not always an option, especially in advanced cases. Once again, there are some antipsychotics that are more appropriate than others in Lewy body disease.

The anti-psychotic issue and Lewy body disease is so critical that we should have our first discussion of specific medications here. As discussed, all Lewy body patients, whether suffering with PD or DLB have low levels of dopamine. We also know that anti-psychotic drugs block dopamine obviously making them a terrible class of drugs for Lewy body patients. But, we also now understand that Lewy body diseases are often associated with severe psychosis, particularly visual hallucinations. In many cases there are no other options but to use anti-psychotic drugs when considering the over-all treatment picture and quality of life.

If required, Seroquel (quetiapine), or Abilify (aripiprazole) are always the first line choices. They tend to be much less harsh in their dopamine blockade and in many cases are actually well tolerated without side effects. Zyprexa (olanzapine) and Clozaril (clozapine) may be second line options but these can be very problematic drugs as we shall see later. High potency anti-psychotics like Risperdal or haloperidol are very useful in dementia in general but will not be well tolerated by Lewy body patients and should be avoided. The result could be extreme Parkinson symptoms that are potentially lethal. There is evidence that patients with Lewy body disease respond well to other medications such as anti-depressants or cholinesterase inhibitors however they may not address the severe psychosis seen in this illness. Of course, medications in general should be avoided if possible and we shall see how they may be minimized in many cases. We shall discuss the anti-psychotics and all other drugs in more detail as well later.

Chapter 5

Other dementias

Alzheimer's disease, Vascular Dementia, and Lewy Body related dementia probably encompass some eighty to ninety percent of all dementias. There are, however, many other types. Many of these are found in younger adults as well as the elderly. In this chapter we shall review the most common of these.

Alcohol (Ethanol) dementia

If there is a fourth most common form of dementia it may well be related to alcohol. This under-rated form of dementia may go undiagnosed for some time due to the relatively younger population it occurs in and their ability to hide their confusion. This "confabulation" is classic alcohol dementia and is more commonly known to clinicians as Korsakoff's psychosis.

Alcohol is a brain toxin that is commonly and voluntarily used by the general adult population throughout the world. There are a variety of confusional states related to alcohol consumption. The dementia is only the end result of years of abuse and generally many bouts of other forms of related confusion either from actual intoxication or withdrawal. Not uncommonly alcoholics develop the Wernicke encephalopathy. This is a potentially reversible acute confusion state caused by a thiamine (vitamin B1) deficiency. Due to their limited diet, this is common to severe alcoholics. It usually responds well to replacement therapy with thiamine. For this reason, alcoholics presenting to an emergency department are usually started on100mg of thiamine daily. The classic Wernicke encephalopathy (encephalo – brain, pathy – disease) involves a traid of symptoms used to identify it: confusion, gait disturbance (ataxia), and a wandering eye (ophthalamoplegia). Each aspect of the syndrome may be present in varying degree.

Unfortunately, Wernicke's encephalopathy is often associated with some degree of the incurable Korsakoff's psychosis. As noted above, Korsakoff's is actually a dementia that may or may not involve psychosis and always involves an element the unique feature of confabulation. Such patients attempt to bluff their way around examining questions in an attempt to hide their confusion. But this "bluffing" is hardly intentional. The unique feature of the damage from alcohol seems to create a state, perhaps layered upon years of lying and denial, of unbelievable storytelling. An inexperienced listener may be taken in and not recognize the degree of confusion. Those with experience however will immediately note that something is not right. Putting the picture together with the history of alcoholism and the lack of any other explanation may well lead to a diagnosis of Korsakoff's psychosis. The condition is likely permanent.

Street drug dementia

The chronic use of street drugs and substances has been thought to cause dementia-like states as well. Many descriptions have been used to identify such conditions such as, frying one's brain, being burnt out on drugs, and having brain rot. While there is no firm evidence that drugs like marijuana, heroin, or LSD cause dementia, there are certainly "soft" psychological profiles that seem regularly associated with the chronic user and may have some organic basis. On the other hand, angle dust (PCP), solvents, and glue present such radical biologic challenges to the brain that they do seem to cause dementia with the classic memory loss and confusion. Cocaine and amphetamine are difficult to characterize relative to dementia as the user is often forced into a periods of abstinence and apparent recovery due to the radical nature of the addiction and inability to sustain the abuse for long periods of time without other complications such as stroke, heart attack, suicide or murder.

Picks Disease and Frontal-Temporal Dementia

If there is an Alzheimer equivalent for thirty and forty year olds it is a relatively uncommon dementia known as Pick's disease or Frontal-Temporal Dementia (FTD). There are actually subsets of these illnesses but for our purposes we shall consider them all together. The diagnosis is usually made through recognition of the early age of onset of confusion and the characteristic atrophy or shrinkage of the frontal and temporal lobes of the brain leaving the rest of the brain intact. I will never forget my first case. It was the Roosevelt Hospital in New York. The thirty year old daughter in law of a very prominent person in American society presented with weeks of personality change and confusion. We thought initially it had to be drugs. But the entire work-up turned out to be negative....except for the prominent loss of brain in the frontal and temporal lobes on the CAT scan. The diagnosis of Picks disease was made. I did not follow up but she likely died before she was forty as the disease is usually fatal within five to ten years. The cause is unknown. Typical initial symptoms of FTD are personality changes rather than the dramatic memory loss seen in Alzheimer's disease.

Multiple Sclerosis

Multiple Sclerosis is a common neurological disease of white matter that doesn't generally affect cognitive abilities until the advanced stages. The dementia is often obscured by a chronic debilitated physical condition. There is a much higher incidence of Multiple Sclerosis in the northern latitudes. The reason for this is not well understood. One born in the north that moves to the south carries with them a lifetime higher risk of developing the disease. The cause of Multiple Sclerosis is unknown.

Progressive Supranuclear Palsy

Progressive Supranuclear Palsy (PSP) is a severe neurological disease that may involve a variety of movement symptoms as well as a rapidly progressing dementia. Typically there is rigidity about the center axis of the patient with an upward gaze. Like most of these illnesses it is always fatal. The cause is not well understood and treatment is general focused upon comfort.

Huntington's disease

Some dementias have very clear genetic links. One classic in this category is Huntington's disease. We all have two sets of each type of genes. Each type is slightly different from others of the same type in another person as it was ever so slightly modified by our ancestry. Each set came from one parent who in turn got two sets of genes from their parents. There is a 50:50 chance that the father of a child will pass on each lightly modified gene type from either his mother or from his father. Similarly, there is a 50:50 chance of the mother passing on the same but slightly modified gene that she got from either her mother or from her father. One can see therefore, if one parent had one badly modified gene that they had gotten from either parent, the offspring would have a 50:50 chance of getting that gene too.

Huntington's disease is an autosomal dominant disease that is clearly coded for on one specific gene. In order to get this gene (barring a rare mutation) you must have a parent with this gene. The Huntington's gene will always dominate over the normal gene passed on from the other parent. In other words, if one inherits the Huntington gene type they will get the disease - there are no carriers. Obviously, then, the parent who passed on the gene must have the disease. Not quite. This disease does not generally present with symptoms until the thirties or forties, long after many have past on the gene to their children. There is currently genetic testing available but despite this, many with a Huntington parent do not get tested. The reasons are multifactorial ranging from denial to fear to fate or religious belief. Unfortunately, this means that this illness will be passed to 50% of their children.

Huntington's disease generally presents with involuntary wave-like movements known as a chorea. This eventually progresses to a devastating picture of complete neurologic dysfunction including dementia. Death generally happens by age fifty.

Wilson's disease

Wilson's disease is a rare but devastating dementia caused by improper copper metabolism. Consideration for this illness should always be given in any healthy person with an early onset dementia. The tell tale sign of the disease is the presence of Kaiser Fleischer rings that form around the iris of the eye. The disease can be confirmed by finding a high serum ceruloplasmin, the protein that binds with copper.

Spongiform Encephalopathy

Also rare and devastating are an interesting group of dementias called the spongiform encephalopathies. These illnesses are also known as the slow virus encephalopathies. The causal agent, actually smaller than a virus, is a glycoprotein known as a prion. These are naturally occurring proteins in our bodies that can undergo mutation into a malignant form. In most cases, the cause of the mutation is unknown. Some of the dementing diseases caused by prions are Creutzfeldt-Jacob (CJD), Gertmann-Straussler-Scheinnker syndrome (GSS), and Fatal Insomnia (FI). There are even less common familial forms of the diseases where a mutated protein is actually passed along in the genetic pool of a family.

Infectious forms of the mutation, that is, those transmitted through ingestion of infected food, have also been described. The most common of these that is exclusive to humans is Kuru. This rare illness was first described in New Guinea where it was shown to be transmissible via cannibalism. Another form of transmissible spongiform encephalopathy is Bovine Foot and Mouth disease or, more commonly, mad cow disease. The true human implications of this devastating animal illness are not known. An outbreak in the United Kingdom of what appeared to be Creutzfeldt–Jacob disease amongst people who might have eaten beef infected with Bovine Foot and Mouth disease created tremendous concerns in the food industry in the late 1990s. Obviously, great lengths have been taken to avoid human inoculation.

While these diseases can have incubation periods of years, death occurs quickly once the symptoms begin. Each illness may have its own particular scenario. For example, Fatal Insomnia always involves a syndrome that literally involves the inability to sleep. While these illnesses may begin subtly with depression, mild confusion, or headaches, they will each ultimately progress to full-blown neurological devastation including dementia within a year. A certain diagnosis can only be made by brain biopsy and examination of the classic sponge-like changes in the brain tissue. A spike wave phenomenon on the electroencephalogram (brain waves) may provide a useful clue.

Human Immunodeficiency Virus dementia

AIDS or Acquired Immunodeficiency Syndrome is an illness caused by the HIV virus. Kaposi's sarcoma, the skin lesion caused by this virus, was first described centuries ago. For reasons that are not entirely clear, the world- wide epidemic of AIDS began in the late 1970s. It was soon discovered that this illness was caused by blood-blood transmission of the virus. Thus, any group engaged in activity allowing for blood contact from others was considered vulnerable. As most are now aware, this illness has caused great devastation in the homosexual and intravenous drug using community. Many do not know that as much or more impact has been made through sexual transmission in the heterosexual population in third world and developing countries.

There are a variety of different criteria for making the diagnosis of AIDS as this disease may affect various systems in the body. The illness commonly involves the neurologic system. This may occur either directly through the effects of the virus itself or indirectly via parasitic infections in the immunocomprimised brain. The direct effects that the virus has on the brain are the cause of the HIV dementia. This dementia is primarily subcortical; therefore apathy, mood instability, and attention deficit are the characteristic psychiatric symptoms rather than memory loss. There is no cure for HIV illness at this time but advances have been made in stabilizing the progression of symptoms. The degree of occurrence of dementia varies from case to case.

Brain Injury

One could argue that stroke or alcohol dementia is a form of recurring brain injury. Typically, however, brain injury is not thought of as a progressive disease as is the case with dementia. Brain injury may certainly involve a clinical scenario that has many of the same elements as dementia but there are good reasons not to discuss brain injury in detail in this context. Firstly, it is a vast subject unto itself. Secondly, recovery is always hoped for and often achieved - unlike most of the maladies we are discussing here. That said, while I would like to treat all such cases as a temporary condition, the reality is that there is often a residual that lasts a lifetime and may involve many of the same aspects of symptom management and long-term care as with dementia patients. Treatments and symptoms vary and the period of recovery may present some of the greatest behavioral challenges. The causes of brain injury include but are not limited to: tumor, hemorrhagic stroke, head trauma and anoxia (lack of oxygen) from drowning or cardiac arrest. It should be noted that brain injury in general is a known risk factor for developing dementia later in life.

Mental Retardation

This is also a subject that may involve many similarities to dementia particularly in terms of treatment and care. Unlike dementia it occurs from birth and is not progressive. Like brain injury, it is a subject unto itself and deserves and entire book to give it its due. The causes of mental retardation are vast and may or may not be genetic in nature. Patients vary greatly in levels of severity and functional ability. Like head trauma, mental retardation is a known risk factor for the eventual development of dementia.

Chapter 6

The Reversible Dementias

In as much as dementia is generally associated with the destruction the neuron, the major functional brain cell that cannot regenerate, one might wonder how there could be such a thing as a reversible dementia. That line of thinking has merit and the "reversible dementias" could probably be better labeled as something else. They may, however, lead to permanent damage and dementia if not properly treated. Let's call them neuropsychiatric syndromes associated with particular medical conditions which evolve slowly and initially involve reversible symptoms that mimic dementia.

The classic reversible dementias are neurosyphilis, hypothyroidism, and vitamin B12 deficiency. There are others that should be mentioned as well. They include: normal pressure hydrocephalus, Wernicke's encephalopathy and severe depression. Let's look at these conditions individually.

Neurosyphilis

Syphilis is a sexually transmitted illness caused by the bacteria Treponema Pallidum. The course of illness is divided into three distinct stages. Primary syphilis is may be identified by an ulceration on the genitalia called a chancre. A positive blood test for syphilis will confirm the diagnosis. Treatment consists of identifying the infected persons and treating them with penicillin. The treatment is highly successful and the illness is usually terminated at this point.

Sometimes the illness is not identified, the chancre heals and life goes on. The bacteria remain however and may not reappear for a year or two at which time a total body rash may occur. This is typical of secondary syphilis. Treatment with penicillin is usually successful. If allowed, to syphilis may progress to the tertiary or third stage. In this stage it is possible for the heart and aorta to become involved leading to serious cardiovascular complications. It is also possible for the central nervous system to become involved. This is neurosyphilis.

Neurosyphilis may involve the spinal cord causing a condition called Tabes Dorsalis. In this case the victim may walk with a "drop foot" type of gait where the feet slap to the floor with each step rather than landing on the heal. The brain may also become involved creating a dementia like condition.

Syphilis was particularly common in the early part of the 20th century. This was a time before antibiotics. Treatment options included doing nothing or taking a course of arsenic. Many did nothing and later developed neurosyphilis. Al Capone, a famous American gangster, was said to have died of neurosyphilis in prison. Nowadays neurosyphilis is rare. It is most commonly seen in immunosuppressed patients such as those with HIV disease. Those with a positive blood test for syphilis, no history of antibiotic treatment and evidence of possible neurosyphilis such as drop foot or confusion require further investigation.

The test for neurosyphilis involves a lumbar puncture (spinal tap) to draw some cerebrospinal fluid and test it for antibodies against the bacteria. A positive test of the cerebrospinal fluid confirms the diagnosis. Treatment recommendations vary but generally speaking oral antibiotics are not an option. Aggressive treatment would involve two weeks of intravenous penicillin. Considering that any chronic infectious condition may cause cellular damage, results of treatment of neurosyphilis vary and full recovery may not always be possible.

Vitamin B12 deficiency

Vitamin B12 is also called cyanocobalamin. This vitamin is required for the synthesis of the nuclear protein in cells. A deficiency of vitamin B12 may involve both the hematologic (blood) and nervous systems. Typically, vitamin B12 deficiency is associated with anemia. The blood cells are usually enlarged; a condition is called macrocytosis or megaloblastic anemia.

Like syphilis, the nervous system dysfunction may occur in the brain, the spinal cord or both. Spinal cord involvement may involve both motor and sensory tracts. For this reason the neurological aspects of vitamin B12 deficiency are sometimes called Combined Systems Disease. It may first present with a sense of pins and needles. Later a loss of sense of vibration and proprioception (perception of pressures) may occur in the lower extremities. Spastic paralysis may also be seen later on. Falls therefore, may become a symptom. The brain involvement involves a progressive state of confusion, paranoia or depression.

Vitamin B12 is absorbed in the gut at the level of the upper intestine with the help of a protein called intrinsic factor. Intrinsic factor is secreted into the gut from the stomach. Most cases of vitamin B12 deficiency are associated with a lack of intrinsic factor. These include the surgical removal of the stomach and a lack of secretion of intrinsic factor called Pernicious anemia. Vitamin B12 deficiency may also occur after removal of the ilium (a part of the small intestine) where it is absorbed. Nutritional lack of vitamin B12 is rare given the wide variety of foods that contain it. One should be on the lookout for older patients with a history of peptic ulcer disease who may have been treated with stomach surgery before the more contemporary medication therapies arrived.

Replacement of vitamin B12 is generally accomplished through a series of monthly intramuscular injections although oral therapy may be useful in some cases. It is important to remember that neurological symptoms of a vitamin B12 deficiency may occur in the absence of anemia. Also, symptoms of the deficiency can occur with a normal serum vitamin B12 level. Getting a methyl malonic acid (MMA) level can make a more accurate measure of the true vitamin B12 level in the body. MMA is always low when vitamin B12 is low. Neurologic response to treatment may be slow and require more than a year.

Vitamin B1 deficiency

Vitamin B1 is also called thiamine. When a dietary deficiency of this vitamin occurs, a condition known as Beriberi may ensue. One of the symptoms of this condition may be confusion and psychiatric changes. In practice, most of the thiamine deficiency seen in the US is in alcoholics. This group tends to have poor nutrition as well as poor metabolism of this vitamin. We have discussed how alcoholics may develop a syndrome caused by thiamine deficiency that is called Wernicke's encephalopathy. Three symptoms are usually required to make this diagnosis: ophthalmoplegia (wandering eyes), ataxia (disturbance in gait), and confusion. For this reason most alcoholics with mental status changes being treated in a hospital will be placed on thiamine 100mg daily.

Hypothyroidism

Thyroid disease may be associated with mental status changes resembling a dementia and is generally reversible. Also called Myxedema Madness, the psychiatric syndrome associated with hypo or low thyroid hormone levels can be quite dramatic. Before the mental status changes occur however, the classic physical symptoms of low thyroid hormone have usually been present for some time. These may include slowed activity levels, course hair, and insensitivity to cold. The "dementia" varies and may present with slowness in thinking or a florid psychosis that may involve an elaborate delusional system filled with plots, conspiracy and deception. Obviously, thyroid testing should be part of any work up for dementia or unexplained psychosis.

A common patient seen for hypothyroid related mental status change is someone already on replacement therapy for thyroid insufficiency who becomes non-compliant with medication. Such patients were often once hyperthyroid and had surgical or chemical ablation of the thyroid as definitive treatment. In such cases replacement hormone must be taken for life. Reversal of the mental status changes due to hypothyroidism may take up to a year after adequate treatment has begun. The last such case I saw was at the Roosevelt Hospital in New York. A woman with a thyroidectomy years before for Grave's disease had gone off her replacement therapy about 6 months before presentation. She thought it wasn't necessary any longer. While babysitting her grandchild, she laced her mouth with Vaseline and swallowed lye in order to prevent the devil from getting to the child through her. She had zero thyroid hormone in her body but made a complete recovery by the next year with treatment with thyroid replacement and antipsychotic medication.

Normal Pressure Hydrocephalus

Every patient being considered for the diagnosis of dementia needs at least one brain scan. It may be either a CAT or MRI scan. While it is useful to have the supporting findings of small vessel disease or atrophy as we have mentioned, the more important reason for the scan is to rule out Normal Pressure Hydrocephalus or NPH. Cerebrospinal fluid or CSF normally exits in and about the brain. In NPH there is an abnormal accumulation of cerebrospinal fluid causing a dilatation of the spaces or ventricles that exist inside the brain.

Most large appearing ventricles are the result of atrophy as commonly seen in Alzheimer's dementia but occasionally it may be NPH. This makes diagnosing NPH through radiographic studies alone difficult. Complicating things further, the classic clinical symptoms seen in NPH are confusion, ataxia, and urinary incontinence. Obviously, these are common findings seen in many forms of dementia as well.

If the findings on the scan and examination are suggestive then a neurologic consultation is recommended. The neurologist may opt for a "test" lumbar puncture to drain some cerebrospinal fluid and see if there is improvement in the gait which may be immediate. The confusion will usually improve after that. If NPH is diagnosed, a permanent shunt may be placed to drain the fluid from the ventricle.

Major Depression

Major depression, the psychiatric term for serious depression, may be mistaken for dementia. The depression may present for the first time in old age, the same period when dementia might be expected. Depression may present with slowed mentation, difficulty with concentration, apparent confusion, and even psychosis. This condition is called "pseudo-dementia" and may appear just like a new case of dementia. Complicating matters, depression is a very common aspect of dementia. For this reason, any new onset cognitive disturbance in the elderly should include both a depression and a dementia screen as part of the management. Whether associated with dementia or not, the depression is usually treatable. Obviously, depression without dementia is the preferred diagnosis. Be aware that the highest incidence of suicide exists in the elderly. Single white males are of particularly high risk.

Anxiety

Anxiety can be associated with a cognitive disturbance if severe enough. Like depression, a new onset of anxiety in the elderly could be an early sign of dementia. One way to differentiate anxiety from early dementia is to administer anti-anxiety medication over a period of time. The confusion associated with pure anxiety will generally improve and stabilize while that associated with dementia may deteriorate to a delirium caused by the medication.

Severe anxiety, depression or psychosis can appear as a state of catatonia characterized as a seemingly awake yet non-responsive mental state. These patients can seem quite demented, as they demonstrate zero memory or cognitive ability. It can be readily differentiated from dementia however by history and a generally good response to anti-anxiety medication. Catatonia associated with dementia may be a very late stage of the disease.

Chapter 7

Delirium

As mentioned previously, there are other types of organic brain disease. We now know that the damage from brain injury or mental retardation may ultimately culminate in a dementia like picture. Both are listed as risk factors for dementia. There is another major category of organic brain disease that must be understood if managing dementia. This is acute brain failure or delirium. Unlike dementia, delirium happens fast. It is commonly reversible however if allowed to mature will culminate in brain death; not in weeks or months but days or even hours. The causes of delirium are vast and may include virtually any medical process that may affect the brain adversely and progress rapidly.

Delirium is important to understand when managing dementia for two reasons. First, most with dementia are older and more vulnerable to any medical process. Secondly, demented brains have been further compromised. There are no more buffers from adversity before failure commences. Thus, delirium may begin in older persons and particularly those with dementia more readily and often due to medical processes that would not affect the mental abilities of a younger or non-demented person.

Delirium is an acute confusional state caused by a disturbance in brain equilibrium. Progression may occur over seconds to minutes to hours or days. Medical textbooks generally describe "clouding of consciousness" as the hallmark sign of delirium. It is true that most cases of delirium will ultimately lead to a clouding of the consciousness, but this is a late stage event. There is often a myriad of earlier psychiatric symptoms and early recognition and treatment is critical.

The specific cause of delirium can be a drug level, a toxin, an infection, a fever, a pressure...a low oxygen level – any adversity that acutely effects the proper functioning of the brain cells. Whatever the mechanism, the outer layers of the brain are affected first. This is protective. The brain stem, the deepest and most primitive layer of the brain is the ultimate target of any delirious process. This is the part of the brain that controls our heart and lungs while we are unconscious or asleep. When that area is compromised, we die. Just before this happens there is one last emergency measure that the brain performs in attempting to save our life and minimize the final blow of the assault. We fall asleep. Anyone who has ever experienced the delirium of acute alcohol intoxication can attest to this. In this case the clouding of consciousness prevents us from drinking further and actually saves our life.

The layers of the brain often affected first involve mood and perception. Thus changes in mood or hallucinations (particularly visual hallucinations) should always be suspected as early delirium. Next, thinking is affected. Decision-making ability and concentration begin to decline. Finally, the motor area is compromised. Speech becomes slurred. Gait begins to stagger.

Consider again the example of acute alcohol intoxication. It starts with a mood disorder, usually a manic syndrome involving loud speech, hyper sexuality, elated mood and inappropriate behaviors. Soon cognitive functions are affected. Fine motor skills deteriorate. The gait becomes disturbed. The speech is slurred. Finally, sedation and we call it a night having no idea how close we came to dying. The next morning we say that will never happen again. But the next weekend, there we are getting delirious again.

The treatment of any delirium involves the identification and treatment of the cause. Most psychiatric medications should be discontinued in the face of delirium although low doses of antipsychotics may be useful in managing any associated agitation or psychosis. Common causes of delirium in the elderly are listed below. One can see that medication related causes of delirium are very common. Note that, while any medication may cause delirium under the right circumstances, properly prescribed modern psychiatric medication is not a usual cause with the exception of the sedative hypnotics. Delirium may result as a cumulative effect of multiple medications.

Common medications related to delirium:

> Sedative-hypnotics (benzodiazepines)
>> Valium (diazepam)
>> Ativan (lorazepam)
>> Xanax (alprazolam)
>> Halcion (triazolam)
>
> Pain medication (narcotics)
>> Morphine
>> Percocet (oxycodone)
>> Vicoden (hydrocodone)
>> Fentanyl
>> Oxycontin

> Anticholinergic medications (see cholinesterase inhibitors)
>> Zantac
>> Theophylline
>> Coumadin
>> Lasix
>> Digoxin
>> Hydrochlorothiazide
>> Nefedipine
>> Captopril
>> Codeine

Detrol
Benadryl
Thorazine
Mellaril
Elavil
Sinequan
Imipramine
Desipramine
Paxil
Zyprexa
Clozaril

General Anesthetics

Non-medication causes of delirium:

Infectious
Urinary tract infection
Pneumonia
Sepsis

Chronic Medical Illness
Congestive heart failure
Chronic Obstructive Pulmonary Disease
(COPD)

Metabolic
Dehydration
Sleep deprivation
Post surgical metabolic changes

Chapter 8

Initiating treatment

Early evaluations and screenings specific for the detection of dementia are not nearly as common as they should be. Often, an astute examiner seeing a patient for another medical problem will pick up the memory loss on examination. It is estimated that only 20% of cases of early dementia are recognized. Given the likelihood of patient and family denial, months and even years can go by before anybody close to the patient reports anything. Events often unfold well beyond the initial memory loss before any action is taken. If for no other reason, dementia needs to be detected early because the current medications used to treat dementia work best if started early.

Reasons for the ultimate detection of dementia vary. Very commonly there may be an event such as the death or illness of a spouse. Spouses can unknowingly enable a partner who has slowly become cognitively impaired with dementia. The couple may have adapted their routines and habits to the deficit over time. All goes well until the disappearance of the healthy member of the team. Suddenly the dementia appears as a serious issue once the check writer, the grocery buyer, the anchor is gone.

The now solitary and undetected dementia patient has little time for grieving the loss of their mate. Rather, all energy must be invested in staying afloat and hiding the confusion from the world. At times a person with dementia may be so compromised that they are not aware their mate id gone or has died. There have been cases reported of patients living for weeks in feces next to a decaying dead spouse only to die of starvation themself.

One might ask how a healthy spouse could allow their confused companion to progress so far without any intervention. Imagine having gotten married at age eighteen, straight into the relationship from the nest with little or no life experience as an adult. Then, after sixty years of marriage, your mate begins to fade and become confused. Your fear of being alone may be tremendous, as you have never been in the world alone before. Anticipating a potential separation, denial takes over and concerns about the spouse's confusion are kept secret. Ironically, an early intervention would more likely be the scenario that leads to more time together.

Patients with dementia rarely report their own memory loss to doctors. Most such reports come from people with normal memory loss for age. As we age, we will all sooner or later jokingly acknowledge that our memory just isn't what it used to be. But early dementia is no joke. The patient is often anxious and inwardly desperate. They will seldom confide within themselves, let alone a caregiver. It is as though they sense an impending tidal wave.

Psychiatric symptoms are very common in early dementia. Imagine the anxiety and depression that one encounters in isolating themselves from others for fear of embarrassment. Then there is the desperation of staying oriented and not becoming lost in the confusion. Psychosis may eventually enter the picture as the interpretation of the world becomes skewed and oblique. The daughter is recognized as the mother. The current residence is the old farm. A family member's attempt to help may be mistaken as a plot or conspiracy. And so there is further resistance. There is more isolation.

Intervention can in fact be so delayed and behaviors can get so out of control that the initial visit with the doctor could be a family seeking a competency opinion for legal purposes or maybe even looking for involuntary commitment for treatment. States laws vary with regard to these issues. Some are conservative while others are quite liberal. In New York State for example, two licensed physicians and a family member or hospital administrator may have someone committed for any reason as long as they feel the patient would benefit from involuntary treatment. On the other side of the country, in Washington State, doctors have no say in the decision to commit involuntarily. Also, it is important to understand that the word competence is generally a legal term. Only a judge can make that decision in a court hearing. A doctor, or anyone else for that matter, can give an opinion about someone's capacity to make sound decisions. A judge when making a determination about competency often uses these opinions.

In some cases it may be necessary to arrange a visit from mental health nurse or social worker to the home. These services can be sought through the social service department at many hospitals. Many areas have an Adult Protective Service (APS) agency that may initiate an investigation if such visits are denied by the patient. Such visits may provide a variety of functions ranging from ensuring compliance with medication and doctor visits to the acquisition of information for a court to order or intervention.

The reality is that many with dementia can be kept stable at home for quite some time. In the perfect world, involved families would talk openly about issues and bring their elderly loved ones to a caring and experienced geriatric doctor for a complete evaluation of their physical and mental heath. Appropriate doses of medications and recommendations for activities would be prescribed and fully complied with by the patient. The family would sit down and have a long, enthusiastic and meaningful meeting about the living arrangement that would be the most beneficial. It happens but not often enough.

More commonly, bits and pieces of this puzzle are addressed over time as the problems present themselves. The family members experience frustration. They are called upon to be strong, creative and many other things they may not be. There may be an event requiring a medical or psychiatric illness hospitalization.

Chapter 9

The evaluation of dementia

Regardless of how one arrives to the health care provider, it is crucial that a proper diagnosis be made and treatment started. There is no blood test for the most common forms of dementia. The diagnosis is based upon history and examination although may be supported by certain blood tests or radiographic (X-ray) evidence. The psychiatric and neurologic history and examination are of particular interest. Eventually, other issues such as other medical problems and social concerns will need to be addressed as well.

Neuro-psychiatric History

Short-term memory loss is generally considered the hallmark of Alzheimer type dementia. Often times however, the memory dysfunction is not the predominant clinical feature that is reported. This is surely the case with other forms of dementia such as Parkinson's dementia. Social isolation, guardedness, depression, insomnia, and irritability are all quite common. Obviously, these may also be features of other psychiatric syndromes such as major depression, alcohol abuse or anxiety. It is therefore important to understand the nature of dementia relative to onset and course. Typically, any new psychiatric symptom in an elderly person who has no significant prior psychiatric history should be suspicious for either dementia or delirium.

As we have seen, delirium is historically distinguished from dementia by its sudden appearance. One exception to this could be the sharp progressions seen in vascular dementia. Other neurologic syndromes should be ruled out as well by obtaining any history of previous organic brain disease including family history, mental retardation or any history of brain injury.

Bipolar illness and, in particular, schizophrenia do not generally begin in the elder years. While depressive and anxiety disorders do commonly occur in the elderly, there is often either a prior history of them or some new precipitating circumstance. One should be aware that dementia typically causes a sort of expansive characterization of the person's personality. Therefore, any increase in prominent aspects of a personality style such as hoarding, paranoia or dependence should be suspect as possible early dementia.

Medical History

The medical history may contain important information that supports a diagnosis of dementia. One may find a history of non-compliance with medication or unaddressed medical issues as a sign of disorganized thinking. A lack of ability to give a detailed medical history is typical of the patient with dementia who is reporting alone. Those with vascular dementia generally will have a history of diabetes, hypertension and\or atrial fibrillation. Other dementia-like syndromes may be related to HIV disease, alcohol, and syphilis. One must take care therefore to look for signals of substance abuse, sexual promiscuity or other contributors to the various forms of dementia.

As we have seen genetics may play a role in dementia. 10% of Alzheimer's disease cases may have an early onset form of the disease passed on from generation to generation. 50% of a Huntington's patient's children will have the disease. A good medical history is also helpful in assessing one for possible delirium. A recent surgery, medication change, urinary or respiratory symptoms are common. Pain may also be a contributor to new onset depression, anxiety or agitation.

Social History

Those with dementia may come from any ethno-geographic background, social-economic level, or have any educational-occupational history. Obviously, an elderly person who is isolated, unable to care for him or herself, or living in an untenable sanitary situation should raise suspicion. Certainly a history of alcohol abuse may be significant, as would IV drug abuse and history of promiscuous sex as it relates to HIV disease and syphilis.

Special education or slow learning is often part of the history of those with retardation or developmental disorders. Such patients commonly do not marry and spend a great deal of their lives doing menial jobs while living at home or under the care of others well into adulthood. Mental retardation is very commonly confused historically with schizophrenia. Schizophrenics, however, do not generally have any history educational problems prior to the late teens and will often have required years of high doses of anti-psychotic medication to control their symptoms. Industrial exposure may be the cause of organic brain disease and a dementia like syndrome. This explanation is often considered by families to be the cause of an otherwise unexplained dementia. While this may be a contributor to the disease, a purely industrial caused dementia is relatively rare from my experience.

Mental Status Examination

The definitive part of the physical assessment that best evaluates a patient for dementia is a specialized aspect of the neurologic examination called the mental status examination. In essence, this is the specialized part of the physical examination used by psychiatrists to do their assessment. This examination, corroborated by the history, is crucial in making the diagnosis of dementia since there is often no definitive test. Let's take a look at the typical aspects of a psychiatric examination.

General appearance and dress
Abnormal movements or tremor
Level of alertness
Orientation to person, place, and time
Short and long term memory
Mood
Affect or relatedness
Level of anxiety
Thought content - delusions, paranoia, obsessions
Thought process - tangential or scattered thinking
Perceptions - hallucinations
Presence of suicidal or assaultive thoughts

We have seen that dementia may present not just with a memory or cognitive deficit but also paranoia, depression or anxiety. Clearly, putting a complete mental status examination in context with the history is the definitive manner to make a certain dementia diagnosis. It remains the case however, that most cases of dementia will present with some degree of memory or cognitive deficit. These aspects of the examination should be of particular interest when suspicious about dementia. Lets look a typical method of conducting this part of the examination.

Orientation
What is the date?
Where are we?
Who am I?

Cognition
Spell the word WORLD forwards and
backwards
What is 100-7, 93-7, 86-7…

Memory

> Repeat the names of three objects
> Repeat the names of the same objects after three minutes
> What did you have for breakfast?
> Who is the president?
> Who was president before that?

Long-term memory may well be preserved in dementia however short term memory is disturbed in most cases. In advanced cases, time and place are diminished as well as other cognitive abilities. Remember that other non-Alzheimer dementias such as vascular, Parkinson or Lewy Body can initially present with deficits in cognitive areas other than memory such as a slowing of mental processing, decreased attention span, and problems with visual-spacial recognition.

Mini-Mental Status Examination (MMSE)

Because the vast majority of people with dementia have some degree of memory or cognitive deficit, the focus is primarily on these aspects of the mental status when screening for dementia. In most instances the mini-mental status examination (MMSE) is used. The mini-mental status examination is a standardized way of performing the cognitive part of the mental status examination that we just reviewed. By standardizing the examination, one can have reliability between different examiners and a standard reference to refer back to on future examinations. It is an easy test to train staff to perform and is relatively quick, non-threatening and painless. The mini-mental status examination can be very useful therefore in monitoring the advancement of the disease and the response to certain treatment strategies. It has been very useful to pharmaceutical companies in assessing their new dementia medications. The test is scaled on a point system from 0 to 30 with a result of less than 26 being suspicious for dementia:

The Mini-Mental State Exam

Patient_____ Examiner

_____ Date_____

Maximum Score

Orientation

5 ( ) What is the (year) (season) (date) (day) (month)?

5 ( ) Where are we (state) (country) (town) (hospital) (floor)?

Registration

3 ( ) Name 3 objects: 1 second to say each. Then ask the patient

all 3 after you have said them. Give 1 point for each correct answer.

Then repeat them until he/she learns all 3. Count trials and record.

Trials _____

Attention and Calculation

5 ( ) Serial 7's. 1 point for each correct answer. Stop after 5 answers.

Alternatively spell "world" backward.

Recall

3 ( ) Ask for the 3 objects repeated above. Give 1 point for each correct answer.

Language

2 ( ) Name a pencil and watch.

1 ( ) Repeat the following "No ifs, ands, or buts"

3 ( ) Follow a 3-stage command:

"Take a paper in your hand, fold it in half, and put it on the floor."

1 ( ) Read and obey the following: CLOSE YOUR EYES

1 ( ) Write a sentence.

1 ( ) Copy a design shown.

_____ Total Score

ASSESS level of consciousness along a continuum

_____

Alert Drowsy Stupor Coma

Neurologic Examination

Other aspects of the neurological status may be useful in assessing a patient who may have dementia. Of great importance is the level of alertness. Those with dementia may be quite blunted or flat in their relatedness or affect but are generally not lethargic by virtue of the dementia alone. This is often a sign of delirium. A diagnosis of delirium may be further supported by a stooping posture, slurred speech, staggering gait and weakness.

Strokes are often associated with dementia. Common findings in a new stroke may be a delirium. Later there is often a focal finding such as a paralysis on one side. A right-sided paralysis means a left sided stroke because of the crossing over of the nerve fibers on their path down to the spine. The left side of the brain is usually where the speech center is. Therefore, it is very common for one with a right side paralysis to have a speech impediment. This is known as aphasia. Aphasia may be of the motor type where it's hard to get the right words out or receptive where it's hard to understand words of others. As you might imagine aphasia can make the assessment of dementia difficult.

Movement disorders or tremor are found in some dementias. A slow frequency tremor is usually present in Parkinson's dementia and may be present in Lewy Body dementia. A rhythmic movement known as a chorea is present in Huntington's disease.

While most cases of dementia will ultimately be associated with ataxia or trouble walking, we have already seen that some are specifically linked to this this from early on. These include Parkinson's dementia, vitamin b12 deficiency, alcohol related Wernicke's encephalopathy, neurosyphilis, and normal pressure hydrocephalus.

Eye findings specific to some dementia include a gaze disturbance sometimes seen in alcohol dementia, progressive supranuclear palsy, and the Kaiser-Fleisher rings around the iris in Wilson's disease of copper metabolism.

Physical Examination

Relative to dementia a complete physical examination should be performed for three reasons:

1. Specific physical findings are helpful in establishing a diagnosis of certain dementias. These include hypertension and atrial fibrillation in vascular dementia, evidence of liver disease in alcohol dementia, and Kaposi's sarcoma or pneumonia in HIV dementia.
2. Patients with dementia are at risk for falls, trauma and bedsores. They are not always able to point out physical problems or pain in the history.
3. Patients with dementia are often unable or unwilling to maintain their medical health. The initial examination is often an opportunity to stabilize known old problems and identify knew ones.

Blood Tests

Most blood tests are ordered in the interest of establishing medical stability. Some will help to establish a cause of delirium. There is no specific test for the most common types of dementia however it is often important to rule out less common types if there is reason to believe they exist. Some of the routine blood tests include the following:

1. CBC – red and white blood cell count to assess anemia and infection.
2. BMP – basic metabolic panel includes electrolytes, acid base assessment, kidney/hydration status, and glucose.
3. LFTs - liver functions assess liver for disease
4. Vitamin B12 – rule out B12 deficiency
5. TFTs – thyroid functions assess thyroid status
6. RPR, FTA or VDRL – tests for syphilis

Tests specific for some less common dementias include:

1. Huntington's disease genetic testing – will specifically tell if patient has gene for HD.
2. Ceruloplasmin – will rule out Wilson's disease of copper metabolism
3. HIV testing – will help establish diagnosis of HIV dementia

Other tests that may help establish the presence of delirium include:

1. Toxicology – identify the presence of a toxic substance
2. O2 saturation – establish blood oxygen level

A likely genetic link to Alzheimer dementia is the APO-E4 test. The significance of this test was discussed earlier.

Urine Tests

A simple urinalysis is fundamental in the early detection of delirium. Any infection in the elderly, especially in someone who is already confused from dementia can cause substantial delirium. The most common is a urinary tract infection (UTI). The symptoms can sometimes be subtle or not elicited by history however. UTIs are more common in females because the anatomy affords easier access of the bacteria into the urethra and bladder. Obtaining an uncontaminated sample of urine however is much more difficult in a female. Nurses may perform a simple catheterization to obtain a valid specimen. Unlike feces, normal urine is sterile. Urine toxicology is another way to screen for some intoxicating substances.

Radiology (X-Rays)

One of the most popular but perhaps over rated tests used for the evaluation of dementia is the CAT scan (computerized axial tomogram) or its newer cousin the MRI scan (magnetic resonance image). The reason behind the popularity is obvious – there's a problem in the brain and a scan shows a picture of the brain. It really is quite remarkable to look at a CAT scan as one does see a virtual picture of sections or slices of the brain as thought it were laid out for examination.

The primary reason for obtaining a CAT or MRI scan of the brain should be to rule out treatable conditions that present as a dementia or a change in mental status. Unfortunately, these scans are only supportive in making the diagnosis of common types of dementia and must be viewed in relation to the clinical picture. Listed below are common abnormal findings related to dementia on CAT and MRI scans that may be seen:

Non-treatable findings

1. Diffuse atrophy – shrinkage of brain seen in Alzheimer's dementia. This is also a normal finding in the elderly.
2. Frontal/temporal atrophy – specific atrophy seen in frontal-temporal dementia (Picks disease)

3.   Peri-ventricular white matter ischemic changes or small vessel disease – may be microscopic strokes but the clinical significance has not been determined
4.   Lacunar infarcts – specific small strokes that may be related to dementia
5.   Old infarcts – old larger strokes that may be related to dementia
6.   White matter plaques – commonly seen in multiple sclerosis

Potentially Treatable Findings

1.   Diffuse cerebral edema – swelling of the brain is an early response to any massive assault on the brain whether traumatic, infectious or metabolic. This is a catastrophic emergency that may in itself cause death.
2.   New cerebrovascular accident (CVA) – a new stroke commonly presents as a specific area of edema. It may be bleeding or hemorrhagic. Specific treatment to the injured brain tissue must be started within hours of symptoms.
3.   Intercerebral or subarachnoid bleed – non-stroke bleeding in the brain is usually caused by a bleeding blood vessel or trauma
4.   Brain tumor – may be benign or malignant. Frontal lobe tumors may present with psychiatric symptoms.
5.   Enlarged ventricles – may be normal pressure hydrocephalus (NPH) but more likely just atrophy. This must be correlated with clinical picture of confusion, ataxia and bladder incontinence.
6.   Subdural hematoma – bleeding between skull and brain may be associated with trauma from a fall.

7. Brain abscess – may be found in IV drug addicts and AIDS patients

Lumbar Puncture (spinal tap)

There are certain conditions that may present as a change in mental status with helpful diagnostic findings in the cerebrospinal fluid (CSF). The CSF is the fluid that surrounds the brain and flows down the spinal column below the level where the spinal cord frays into individual nerves in the lower back. A sample of fluid can therefore be safely obtained with a needle from the lower back. The most common indications for a lumbar puncture are listed below:

1. Meningitis/cerebritis – any change in mental status associated with an unexplained fever may represent an infection in the central nervous system
2. Neurosyphilis – a newly diagnosed dementia with a positive blood syphilis test may represent neurosyphilis. In neurosyphilis the CSF tests positive for syphilis just as the blood did.
3. Alzheimer's dementia (experimental) – it is only a matter of time before specific proteins found to be associated with this most common dementia are available outside the laboratory

EEG (brain waves)

The electroencephalogram is a method of measuring the electrical activity in the brain and may demonstrate various forms of problems. Most commonly abnormal brain waves are used to verify the presence of seizure activity. A generalized slowing of brain waves is commonly seen in dementia. EEG is also commonly used for sleep disorder studies. The EEG is a painless test that involves placement of electrodes on the scalp much like that of EKG electrodes on the chest. The test does require that the patient lie still for a period of time.

Amytol Interview

Sensationalized by the movies, there is an accepted medical procedure where a drug is used to intoxicate an individual to gain information. This procedure is known as the Amytol interview. While sodium amytol is most commonly used, sodium pentothal is the drug better known to Hollywood and us. The general idea is simple - sedate a person enough with a hypnotic medication to where they become disinhibited and begin to tell what is really on their mind. There should be nothing mysterious about this procedure as it happens every night at the local corner bar or tavern.

In practice however, the purpose of the test is not really about gaining specific information. In certain cases a patient may present in a catatonic state where they are awake but not responding. The cause of such a condition is usually either organic brain disease or a psychiatric trauma commonly known as a dissociative state. An Amytol interview is sometimes necessary to differentiate the two. The psychiatric patient should come out of the catatonia briefly and be more responsive. A patient with dementia or delirium will generally drift deeper into cerebral depression and fall asleep.

Chapter 10

The early stage of dementia

The management of each case of dementia is a long-term endeavor that will be in a constant state of evolution. Medical problems will arise, and medications, both medical and psychiatric, will change or be adjusted. Living situations will evolve towards provision for more and more structure. And the more structure, the higher the expense. In this chapter we shall take a practical look at the early stage of dementia and the different issues that might arise. This is often a silent stage where denial and avoidance win the day. Feelings of anticipation and fear are felt by both patient and family but often not yet shared. This disconnect can lead to isolation and an under treatment of both the dementia and the psychosocial issues surrounding it.

By adulthood we have developed psychologically to the point of being able to have mature relationships with one another. Imagine if things started back the other way. Acceptance of this is the core of the crisis that is the first stage of dementia. Let's consider then, the beginning of the trip backwards where both family and patient are first confronted with the changes. As with any beginning, there are usually more questions than there are answers.

In essence the retrogression of dementia is a separation. For the patient it is a separation from the world. For the family it is a separation from the patient. The struggle is often silent; each party unaware of what they are feeling let alone the other. This is the core of denial. It leads to resistance of treatment as well as a delay in the management of important day-to-day living concerns and frustrations. This may very rapidly translate into a prolonged depression or anxiety disorder in either the patient or family member. Previously mutual social events are now less commonly attended due to anxiety about memory loss, disinterest, or even embarrassments from inappropriate behaviors. The end result for the patient is more time isolated staring at the television or doing solitary activities. This will lead to the spouse having to adapt and spend more time alone doing the activities that used to be done jointly. Importantly, this adaptation on the part of the spouse is often difficult and may even necessitate a therapeutic intervention.

When common time is shared, there comes more and more interpersonal differences and often-increasing disagreement. As the dementia progresses the spouse or family members will realize they are becoming caregivers and the responsible party. The new authoritarian arrangement will be met with rebellion and further disagreement requiring even more restraint and understanding on the part of the healthy companion.

As the divergence progresses between the two parties, questions begin to arise. What about driving? What about the financial decisions? The caregiver will need to assume more and more of these responsibilities. This may not be an important issue for a caregiver who always assumed these responsibilities anyway. It will, however, be a huge if not impossible task for someone who never did these things. And what about alcohol use, socializing or just having fun? For all patients there will be some areas of conflict. Just as with teenagers, no game plans rulebooks are sent out explaining how to deal with these issues. But they are serious and could eventually jeopardize the health or welfare of someone.

Creativity is usually required in the early stages of dementia. Perhaps an allowance for a glass of wine here and there or some supervised bill paying gives just enough sense of purpose and control to the patient as to calm the storm. Things will change as the illness progresses. Adjustments will be necessary with greater demand for more creative and gentle ideas. Confrontation too must be done with care and thought. Harsh confrontation will only be met with the same rebellion one might expect from a teen. At the same time however, firm limits must be set before danger occurs. Again, the pre-dementia situation may well determine how much of an issue this is. If the spouse with dementia was dependent and easy going it might be easy. However, imagine the situation where the dependent one is the healthy caregiver and the domineering one is getting progressively more rebellious and confused. Consider too, that personalities do on occasion change with the onset of dementia. A previously calm personality may turn mercurial.

There are an infinitesimal number of issues that might come up but some commonalities. Interpersonal problems with dementia are most intense at home. Consider that an early response to memory loss and confusion is to physically isolate oneself from public and be at home more often. Stress may build in the home as conflicts develop. Lurking behind the scenes we find denial making it impossible to confront the issues because nobody knows, wants to talk about, or wants to hear why this is all happening in the first place.

But why would there be such denial? Well, in the first place, dementia is subtle in the beginning. These are changes that are hard to notice and are issues that don't want to be noticed; they are always placed on a back burner. Of course, from a spouse or family perspective the slow and agonizing loss a loved one is difficult to accept. It is often easier to adapt and look the other way. Sadly, this is a moment when there is an illness to diagnose and treatment plans to be developed. Some treatments such as cholinesterase inhibitors are always best started early.

Dedication and loyalty are reasons for denial too. Spouses will fight for the integrity of their loved one until the end no matter how hard the caregiving becomes. And there is one other reason for denial that is specific to the spouse. Imagine being married to someone at age eighteen. You spend the next sixty years together and then over the course of that sixtieth year comes the dementia. The spouse and soon to be caregiver is facing being alone for the first time in their life. Desperation sets in. This may be a point fir the healthy partner where loyalty and fear may begin to merge. Only by examining these issues openly can one proceed forward and make sound decisions, maintain a safe and stimulating environment, and plan for future.

The following are healthy actions in dealing with early dementia:

1. Get to a doctor and get an evaluation. There is nothing to gain by avoidance. If it is dementia, the sooner you begin to address the issues, the better. If it is not dementia it could be another life threatening illness that needs to be dealt with. The spouse or caregiver needs to deal with his or her own health as well.

2. Whether you are a spouse, family member or just the responsible party, examine yourself from within. Examine your fears and concerns that might interfere with sound decision making for the afflicted person?

3. Get a lawyer skilled in dementia care issues and plan your financial attack. How will you pay for the dementia care? In the US, Medicare will not pay for most dementia care. Medicaid will pay for some. You stand to be forced to accept an inappropriate care situation or lose your life savings if you are not prepared financially.

Chapter 11

The middle stage of dementia

The middle stage of dementia is often considered the worst. The stormy nature of this stage is fueled by the patient's deteriorating condition. Most caregivers have by now become convinced they are dealing with a severe illness and are witnessing the serious decline in the one they love and\or care for. Let's return to the metaphor of traveling through life backwards as the dementia progresses. Imagine going through puberty in reverse. Now stripped of your adult rights to drive and make basic decisions alone, you are faced with losing your basic dignity. To some degree you are aware of the worsening deterioration in your cognitive functioning. You fight tooth and nail to stay afloat and keep your sanity. The mornings are easier despite the fact that you may not have slept well. But there's no time to be tired. You have to convince others that you are okay and are still who you were yesterday morning. But as the afternoon blends into evening, things change. It's like being kidnapped and forced into your past because that's all you remember. The present situation becomes blurred and unreadable. People are no longer who they say they are and you are no longer who you think you are. Suddenly you are underwater and all you see is an image of the farm you may have grown up on. You are with your mother now. You feel better.

The person who is being misinterpreted as the mother may be the patient's sister or wife. They may rub the forehead of the confused person having witnessed a severe transformation in mental state over the past six hours. This transformation phenomenon is known as sundowning. It occurs daily starting in the afternoon and persists into the evening. The experienced caregiver will have accepted the mother role and to some degree even have played into it. They realize from experience that fighting it its fruitless; that it may even be therapeutic to allow the psychosis to emerge. The less experienced caregiver will be distressed by the transformation and fight against the idea that they are misidentified as someone else. This will only lead to distress in both the caregiver and patient.

As you might imagine, there is a good chance that some sort of psychiatric intervention may be necessary in the middle stage of dementia. Psychiatric medications can make enormous improvements however less medication of any kind is always best. They should, therefore, not be used unless behavioral and environmental therapies have been exhausted. Let's look at some of the different ways that experts at a well run assisted living dementia care facility might manage psychiatric issues in the middle stage of dementia.

Behavioral management means addressing aberrant behavior without the use of either force or medication. Medication may have side effects and mix poorly with other medications. The use of force has no place outside of absolute psychiatric emergencies where physical restraint will protect someone from injury. The need for such action is generally a symptom of an unaddressed problem. It is never a viable means for continued caregiving. The use of physical restraint in fact has become a huge area of concern that it is highly restricted in all health care settings. Psychiatric units for example are no longer able to restrain or seclude patients without constant monitoring and documentation of its necessity by doctors and nurses. Nursing homes are virtually unable to restrain unless 911 is being called simultaneously. Even a circumventing walker or sweptback chair where a person is being held back by gravity is considered a restraint and is against many regulations.

So then, what is behavioral management? This is an intervention made by caregivers to curb or change a particular behavior. Generally, a behavior requiring an intervention has been determined to not be in the interest of that person or may endanger someone else. There is a broad range of examples ranging from simple acts like encouraging someone to eat or more serious encounters such as redirecting someone away from a potentially violent situation. Considering all of the laws and regulations against restraint and all the concerns about medications, this is an area of study that has become important to those interested in dementia and long-term care. There are experts who have created systematized styles or methods for dealing with behavior. These can be found in the many books and seminars on the subject and are often adopted by long term care facilities as a standardized way of teaching staff about managing behavior. They often offer extremely useful techniques for all of us who deal with dementia patients. While some techniques may seem born out of an anti-medication position, I would encourage the reader to become informed about all proven methods of improving the quality of life in those with dementia.

Validation, re-direction, and re-orientation are some of the common themes in behavioral management. They are useful because of the ease at which a person with a short-term memory deficit can be induced to think differently or change the stream of thoughts and feelings. Someone who is distressed over confusion may only need to feel accepted to feel calm and less anxious. A stubborn attempt to stay in the wrong room may easily be thwarted by a creative change of focus onto a subject that is of more interest to the patient. And there is nothing like a simple reminder of an appointment that was indeed kept to calm someone who is nervous about missing it because of poor memory. Such methods are very effective, non-toxic, and easy for caregivers to learn.

One limitation of behavioral management is that the effect of these interventions may be short term. A behavioral procedure may well alleviate a dangerous situation. But what if serious potential for the situation to recur still exists? Another problem is a matter of intensity. Some intense beliefs cannot be changed by behavioral means. Certainly, many distorted beliefs need not be changed but what if they are causing distress or are dangerous?

Let's return to the previous example of the female family member or caretaker mistaken as the mother. Such thoughts can eventually expand and include all females. What if this creates agitation or violence every time a female caregiver is encountered? Such a problem will eventually require some sort of resolution - female caregivers are hard to avoid in most caregiving situations. Caregivers must also carefully examine their own reactions to behaviors and make certain they are not treating themselves by extinguishing a behavior that is questionably distressful to a patient.

This touches on the theme of the wandering explorer. It has to do with an acceptance of those stricken with dementia as people still having their persona. This is important because in dementia some level of confusion will be permanent and it will progress. But, behind the confusion and wandering there is a purpose - an explorer. This is an inherent aspect of our human nature that, no matter how off course we may be, we will still be heading somewhere with a purpose, until the end. A daughter once said, "This is not my dad anymore". What if her father had not seen the purpose in her when she was an infant?

It should be pointed out that caregiving with dementia patients can be dangerous. Patients can be physically healthy despite their confusion and more than able to afflict significant injury. Caregivers must learn to recognize situations where behavioral techniques may have limited results and where they may be placing themselves in harms way. Warning signs to be particularly weary of include the following:

And history of violent behavior
A large male patient
Any escalation of emotional intensity

That is not to say that such patients or situations should be avoided. Rather, the following is recommended until a high level of confidence is attained:

Provide care with more than one caregiver
Avoid potential physical entrapment
Initially, maintain some physical distance
Keep your head and face clear of a strike
When approaching, pleasantly grasp the hands in a gesture of kindness
Speak in soft tones with soft themes
Explain everything you are doing
Immediately back away if escalation occurs

Another way of avoiding the use of medication and restraint is though consideration of the environment. As a rule, dementia patients do better in socially stimulating and structured environments. While most will avoid social situations early on, this social anxiety becomes less intense later. At this point the short-term memory is very short and external reality connections are limited. These patients are alert however and the flawed internal thinking machine is still running. And so, internal misguidance becomes the primary source of hope as well as anxiety in the middle stage of dementia. We see their minds wandering but they are reaching, struggling and exploring.

Social stimulation lifts people with dementia from confusion and helps them to track in a reality they can see happening before their eyes. Under stimulation, on the other hand, leaves the patient at the mercy of confusion. It is an exhausting, depressing and anxiety provoking experience to be confused.

While it is certainly possible to over stimulate dementia patients, they have a general tendency to respond well to events and interaction. Having an understanding of the proper quality and quantity of social stimulation for dementia has become a major aspect of dementia care.

Many skilled nursing and assisted living facilities have become sophisticated in creating environments that offer appropriate social stimulation. A major effort is made by the better facilities to provide a pleasant and safe environment with caregivers that take the initiative and engage patients before any problematic behaviors are allowed to develop. Further, many patients may continue to isolate themselves and require encouragement to participate socially. Activities should be continuously available with varying degrees of necessity. These might range from going to the doctor or other health care needs to meals, religion and entertainment activities. All activities are deliberately set up in such a way as to make the experience as enjoyable and stress free as possible. One activity that is commonly missing at many facilities is a therapeutic group specifically designed to provide a place where patients can share experiences and hear about those of others. This is a perfect situation to observe early signs of trouble such as depression, increased confusion or physical pain.

It requires considerable effort to create acceptable environments for dementia care. While many families and spouses are successful at attaining this at home, most will agree that the energy required in doing so can be overwhelming. Life would be optimal if it could all be done at home. The cost is usually less, the environment and caregivers are familiar, and the family has closer control. Yet the assisted living and adult family home business is thriving. The reasons for home failure vary. I have listed some of those I see as being most common:

Family or spouse unavailable for caregiving
Behaviors unmanageable at home
Medical care unmanageable at home

Whether at home with the spouse or in a facility, creative care should be taken to understand the patient amidst their confusion and what their interests may be. This is often based on past occupations and hobbies. Some patients will require more or less independence in their endeavors based on the degree of dementia and their personality style. In the end, environmentally protected patients will be on less psychiatric medication and generally be more fulfilled. This group will also be healthier from a physical standpoint. Every effort should be made to get these patients out of bed and walking. If they cannot walk alone, they should be assisted to on a daily basis by a therapist. This is an exercise that will limit bedsores, lower extremity and pulmonary blood clots and infections like pneumonia.

In due course, there will be encounters with personality issues just as there is with any of us. As a rule, personality styles become more pronounced in the face of dementia. A chronically pessimistic patient will have a serious depression during the course of their dementia. An obsessive type might be a hoarder. A self-centered or narcissistic person will likely get paranoid. Understanding who a person is psychologically will further lessen the chance they will need medication. Ironically, many spouses don't even begin to consider who their spouse really is until they become demented.

There is, of course, another group of personalities we must deal with – us, the children caregivers. Our own neuroticism, in part determined by the demented parent we are caring for, is both a virtue and a curse. It is the resulting conflict between who we were biologically determined to be and who our parents enabled us to be through our relationship with them. It is the psychological fingerprint of who we are individually. It is our flag and our agony. The children are often called upon to make crucial decisions regarding the welfare of a parent with dementia. This can bring up an enormity of issues out of the past because of the reversal in roles. Complicating matters more, there may be siblings involved with differing opinions. Add to this an indecisive spouse, an opinionated friend and the confused patient; you can imagine the mess. Then this mess walks through the front door of the doctor's office, broadsiding the doctor and creating an explosive drama where everyone gets off track. Remember, many physicians are not trained or able to deal with confusing family dynamics.

The following are a list of three major factors to consider relative to the middle stage of dementia:

1. Each patient with dementia will do better if their illness and confusion is accepted and understood by the family and friends who interact with them.

2. People with dementia do better in safe and socially stimulating environments that are creative, employ behavioral techniques and account for personality idiosyncrasies.

3. An appointed lead family member with one capable primary doctor, in consultation with others involved, do best in helping the patient make his or her best choices.

Chapter 12

The late stage of dementia

Generally speaking, dementia is a debilitating illness that will terminate in death after five to ten years. The focus in the final stage of treatment begins to shift from behavioral management to more basic and physical concerns. Those in the late stage of dementia may be no longer able to feed themselves, bathe or toilet themselves. They may not even be able to get out of bed alone. This exposes the patient to a myriad of serious conditions. The killers in dementia are opportunists that prey on chronically immobilized and malnourished individuals with weakened defensive systems. Let's take a closer look at the behavioral issues in this later stage of dementia and explore the medical concerns that ultimately lead to death. We shall see how a stimulating environment continues to be necessary and begin a discussion of "nursing homes" as an option for terminal care.

Most patients with dementia, despite their confusion, will stay psychologically alive until the end. This means that encounters with anxiety, agitation, mood disturbances or psychosis are inevitable. These patients will need closer and closer scrutiny of their psychiatric medication as they become more fragile and vulnerable to delirium. At the same time, however, behavioral management techniques will become less and less reliable as the degree of confusion mounts. This leads one down a narrowing corridor where medication may become more necessary while the likelihood of complications from that medication is more likely. Creative management again becomes a part of getting past such complexities. Let's start to explore some of that creativity first by seeing if there are any advantages to a later stage of dementia.

First, the distorted window into reality that is experienced by a patient will fuel much of their behavioral drama. This is common in the middle stage of dementia. Patients often have a sense of becoming overcome by the confusion between what is real and what is not. This creates a tremendous amount of anxiety, fear and instability throughout the course of the day. Later on however, there are less rubs with reality. The entire world is one of confusion and psychosis, often painted onto a backdrop of memories of events that occurred when the patient was much younger. Certainly, if the patient had a turbulent past, this too can create fear and anxiety but there does seem to be some advantage to being more consistently confused.

Also, when a more physically declined person has behaviors they are less able to mobilize themselves. These weakened patients engage in behaviors that are generally more easily managed.

For any advantages there may be in dealing with a later stage of dementia there are as many disadvantages. As I have said this is a vulnerable and sensitive population. When behaviors do emerge in the later stage of dementia, delirium must always be considered. These patients are often so weak that small amounts of medication, respiratory or urinary tract infections, and even pain can create severe delirium. This may manifest itself with agitation, psychosis, more confusion or a mood disturbance. Lethargy, even stupor may set in as the delirium mounts.

Deterioration and progression of the dementia are inevitable. There comes a point where patients are less able to move around on their own. If no one can help, they may be stuck or alone for long periods. Without walking there is less use of the leg muscles. Blood clots can form and pressure ulcers on the back and feet may appear. The heart and lungs are less exercised. Pneumonia and other opportunistic infections become more likely.

Therefore, one important reason for the stimulating environment is to promote continued mobilization as long as possible. The environment should not only encourage mobility but also allow for safety. This may be the point where purposeful exploration on the part of the patient is at a minimum and aimless wandering becomes the primary mode of activity. Speech may be rambling and unintelligible. Obviously, some limits must be set on certain behavior if it escalates to a dangerous or disruptive level. Decisions must be made between behavioral management that might marginally solve a problem and using medication that might over sedate a very sensitive patient and risk medical complications.

A good reason for a stimulating environment is to limit the amount of medication. I have seen many patients brought into hospital from isolated situations, covered with bedsores, psychotic, unable to engage socially, and on multiple medications. Put into a stimulating environment with proper nutrition, wound care, and social interaction, many such patients can improve dramatically in a couple weeks. They may be walking again, have less confusion, and be of a brighter spirit. It is true that this can bring its own problems such as becoming a fall risk developing a new paranoia as they are now able to think again, but these problems are usually manageable. The alternative would have been death.

Sooner or later those with late stage dementia will die. People at times seem to make a choice to die while others go out with a fight in what has been described as terminal agitation. Social isolation, decreased eating, a lessening of participation with care, and apparent depression are commonly seen at this time. This is certainly a time in the course of treatment where many ethical issues can enter the picture. When is the right time to let a person go? How much pain medication or tranquilization does one give? As such care decisions are made, there are a couple of important things to keep in mind.

First, the time to die may not be right. All patients deserve some consideration of whether or not there is the possibility of some quality of life and happiness that can be attained. This may occur through addressing medical issues, psychiatric issues, nutrition, mobilization, socialization or a combination of all the above. This also serves the purpose of ruling out neglect. Many areas of concern here have been studies extensively. For example, there have been several studies looking at feeding tubes. Unless being used for a situation where recovery is expected, feeding tubes do not improve or extend to its recipient any quality of life. They are often deterrents for socialization from caregivers and a continuous source of infection.

Secondly, no dying patient should have poor hygiene, untreated bedsores, or be denied access to social interaction. This is neglect and any evidence of it should be reported to an adult protective service agency.

Most patients in the terminal stage of dementia will either be at home or in a nursing home. Nursing homes are known today in the US as skilled nursing facilities (SNF). They are not appropriate for all patients with advanced dementia nor are all beds in skilled nursing facilities filled with advanced demented patients. Many patients with advanced dementia are at home. There is a general feeling that home is good. Home is where the heart is. Home is home. But home is not always the best choice or possible in advanced dementia.

Specialty care has now emerged in most skilled nursing facilities. This has come with increased regulations by governments as well as the increased specialty training to care for such patients. Dementia care or rehabilitation is now part of the brand of many facilities. Even the general skilled facilities have specialty training and regulations within their doors. Skilled nursing care is a more hospital like situation than assisted living. Patients have a medical chart and are assigned an attending doctor. The role of doctor involvement in long-term care has become more scrutinized. AMDA or the American Medical Director Association is specific to long term care and is growing annually. The nursing care in skilled nursing is much more advanced as well. There is now a much higher ratio of nurses to patients.

Skilled nursing care is under a much higher degree of scrutiny by all states. Although there are still some marginal facilities, there are few that are bad. Most states have mounted aggressive efforts to shut down facilities that are not up to standards. A list of the state reviews of facilities can be found on the Internet. Assisted living and adult family homes, while scrutinized, have a much lower bar in front of them.

We have reviewed some of the issues particular to the later stage of dementia. In essence this is a time with the potential for complete loss of independence and ultimately, death. Severe medical issues may take precedence but the need for a stimulating environment remains.

Consider these important issues relative to advanced dementia:

1. Understand that there may be increasing need for medical management including hospitalizations due to the fragile nature of these patients.

2. Whatever the living environment, unaddressed bed sores, poor hygiene, or denial of access to social interaction is neglect.

3. Skilled nursing facilities are the ultimate level of care for many with advanced dementia. They are highly

regulated but can vary relative to their ability to give good dementia care. Research them well.

4. Decisions about death and dying are difficult. There may come a time when allowing one to die is the appropriate action.

Chapter 13

Medical issues associated with dementia

There are many medical issues commonly encountered in patients with dementia. While common to the elderly in general, these problems can be lethal to patients with dementia.

Falls

The most common cause of a hip fracture in the elderly is a fall. One quarter of such patients will die within one year. Needless to say, a fall can be devastating. While the most common serious problems associated with falls are fractures, head trauma can obviously be a devastating consequence as well. Falls are more and more common as we age. The muscles in the elderly are weaker and the nervous system is less capable of managing coordinated movement. The circulatory system is less stable and more prone to sudden drops in blood pressure when standing. Combinations of mediations and medical problems may lead to lethargy and a further decline in walking performance.

But it is crucial for the elderly to be as active as possible. Activity, walking in particular, helps to exercise the muscles and circulatory system. The respiratory system is cleansed through exercise thus providing protection against pneumonia. And getting on the feet prevents pressure ulcers from forming on any part of the skin that is continuously abutting a surface.

So, what about patients who are only marginally able to walk? It raises a question that caregivers must deal with – which is worse, the risk of a fall or the risk of pneumonia or a bed sore. There are ways to help with such dilemmas such as walking aides, personal assistance, and physical or occupational therapy but the risks remain.

There are several syndromes associated with ataxia (gait disturbances) and falls that are also associated with dementia and confusion. A few are listed below:

Wernicke's encephalopathy
        Cause – thiamine deficiency
        Symptoms - ataxia, confusion, abnormal gaze
        Suspicion – alcoholism

Combined Systems Disease
        Cause – Vitamin B12 deficiency
        Symptoms – anemia, ataxia, confusion, numbness
        Suspicion – history of upper bowel surgery

Normal Pressure Hydrocephalus
        Cause – Increase cerebrospinal fluid in brain
        Symptoms – confusion, ataxia, urine incontinence
        Suspicion – rapid onset of dementia

Neurosyphilis
        Cause – untreated syphilis infection
        Symptoms – confusion, ataxia, possible heart problems
        Suspicion – history of promiscuity

Pneumonia

Pneumonia is probably the number one cause of death in people with dementia. Pneumonia is an infection of tissue of the lungs. It may be caused by any number of different pathogens from bacteria to viruses to a fungus. While those with chronic long disease such as emphysema or bronchitis are more susceptible, any debilitated person can get it. Specifically, immobility, and aspiration (inhaling your sputum or food) are major causes. Mobilization and preventive swallowing measures such as a diet texture change will help prevent death from pneumonia. Treatment of pneumonia involves identification of the pathogen responsible for the infection and initiation of medication to kill that pathogen. Hospitalization may or may not be required however intravenous fluid is often necessary to prevent dehydration. Intravenous access may also be required for medications in severe cases where a person is unable to take oral medication. Pneumonia is a major cause of delirium in the elderly.

Chronic Obstructive Pulmonary Disease

Also known as COPD, Chronic Obstructive Pulmonary Disease is usually a product of years of smoking cigarettes. COPD is more commonly known as emphysema and bronchitis. The typical course of the illness is a slow and progressive permanent deterioration of the lung tissue (emphysema) with intermittent flare -ups of infection (bronchitis). Unfortunately, quitting smoking after many years is not soon enough for many and they will spend the remainder of their lives dependent upon oxygen, inhalers, and warding off lung infection. Low oxygen levels in the blood can obviously make the confusion of dementia worse. It is a common factor in delirium.

Congestive Heart Failure

If dementia is the clinical syndrome caused by the progressive deterioration of brain tissue then congestive heart failure is that for the heart. Congestive heart failure or CHF is very common in the elderly. Over time the integrity of the heart muscle deteriorates and is no longer able to pump the blood with efficiency. Fluid backs up behind the heart as the result of increased hydrostatic pressure and result in edema or fluid in the tissues. The heart is divided into two distinct sides and the failure may occur more on one side or the other. In left heart failure the fluid will back up in the lungs causing pulmonary edema. This can present with extreme shortness of breath and even gurgling where the patient is literally drowning in fluid inside the lungs. Right heart failure presents with fluid backing up in the gravity dependent areas of the body such as the legs or back depending upon the dominant position of the patient. This is called dependent edema.

While CHF cannot be cured, there are therapies that can be of great help. Digoxin is a medication that will increase of the effectiveness of the heart muscle. Lasix is a powerful diuretic or water pill that will help rid the excess fluid from the body. CHF may present as a medical emergency or be a smoldering chronic condition. Certainly a huge risk factor for CHF is recurrent heart attacks. Prevention of coronary artery disease is therefore crucial to the prevention of CHF. Exercise of the heart muscle and the extremities as tolerated will help to strengthen the heart muscle and squeeze the fluids out of the legs in those with CHF. Unfortunately people with dementia are often immobilized and are at a greater risk for fluid backing up. They often cannot complain of shortness of breath or swollen legs. Great care must be given to monitoring those with CHF and dementia.

Dehydration

In a way, the opposite of CHF is dehydration. In this case, there is too little fluid in the body. The result is a lowering of adequate blood perfusion of critical areas such as the brain. This can lead to a variety of symptoms ranging from weakness to increased confusion or even passing out. The kidney, responsible for fluid management in the body, may shut down in response to dehydration.

The most common cause of dehydration is decreased fluid intake. This commonly occurs in the face of any malnutrition or medical illness where there is a decreased intake. Additionally, medical problems such as pneumonia create a need for excess fluid to fight the infection. In terminal cases, even the management of CHF with Lasix can cause dehydration. As one might imagine therefore, dehydration is very commonly seen in dementia and is a frequent cause of deterioration in mental status. Beyond a basic monitoring of mental status and looking for dry skin texture, trouble with the body's hydration status is confirmed in looking at a kidney function test called the Blood Urea Nitrogen or BUN. Treatment involves replacement of fluid. It may be necessary to do this intravenously. Recovery is usually dramatic.

Urinary Tract Infection

Urinary tract infections or UTIs are common in the elderly. This is particularly so in females because of the anatomic ease at which the bacteria can get inside the urinary tract. Serious urinary tract infections in the elderly are almost always bacterial as opposed to being caused by a virus or fungus. While the offending bacteria may be the same as some infections found in younger people, the presentation is often much different. The brains of the elderly, particularly those with dementia, have an increased vulnerability to systemic toxins released as a result of such an infection.

This means that an infection such as a UTI may present with a change in mental status before any of the classic symptoms such as urine frequency or pain are noted. In fact, in many cases urine symptoms are never noted because someone with dementia may not be able to complain of pain or urine frequency. As a result, those with experience in dementia care know to look for a UTI at the first sign of a change in mental status in a patient with dementia. This change can be anything from a mood swing or agitation to paranoia or a hallucination.

Definitive identification of a UTI is made by obtaining a urinalysis with a culture and sensitivity or UA\CS. Remember, the urine is normally sterile. Obviously care must be taken to get an uncontaminated sample of urine. An antibiotic is sometimes started immediately but the bacteria from the sample should be grown in a laboratory and tested with different antibiotics to confirm sensitivity of the bacteria to the antibiotic that was started. This is called the culture and sensitivity.

As is the case with most infections, if left untreated it will spread though the body and cause sepsis. In the case of a UTI this is caused urosepsis. Sepsis is a medical emergency that if not treated will cause death.

Bed Sores and Ulcers

We who are active take our skin's integrity for granted. One should realize that it is only a short time before a continuous pressure on one part of the skin will begin to cause a breakdown. Obviously this is a common event in the debilitated and dementia patients who are no longer able to mobilize. Those with diabetes are another group that is particularly vulnerable to the development of ulcerations. Common places where this breakdown occurs are the part of the lower back called the sacrum and heals.

Typical stages of the ulcers may range from one to four, as follows:

> Stage I – reddened skin
> Stage II – Blistering or breakdown to the deeper skin layers
> Stage III – Breakdown to the underlying connective tissue
> Stage IV – Breakdown to the underlying muscle or bone

Many with dementia are so confused or have such an impaired sensory apparatus as in diabetic neuropathy that they are not able to report pain associated with the ulcer. For this reason demented patients must be looked over carefully for ulcerations. Early signs of breakdown such as redness are particularly important to look for. Any patient who is in a wheelchair or bed for long periods of time should be treated with preventative measures. These measures include:

> 1) Limiting the amount of time in the wheelchair or bed as much as possible

> 2) Having a regular physical therapy program set up.

> 3) Using heal protectors

> 4) Using an egg-crate mattress or airbed

> 5) Rotating a bed bound person regularly.

The prevention of some ulceration is impossible in those who are permanently disabled. Those that do develop it must be treated aggressively. There are many therapies available and a wound care specialist can best guide appropriate management of a wound. To be sure, if infection has developed, things have gone too far. Sepsis must be managed to prevent a potentially fatal scenario.

Sepsis

We have already seen that sepsis may occur as a complication of infections. Sepsis is an infection that has crept into the bloodstream. It is the result of the spread of a localized infection into the body. It is not uncommon to see sepsis in dementia patients as they are vulnerable to infections and their weakened system will not prevent bacteria from entering to the blood.

Sepsis is a medical emergency and is confirmed by identification of bacteria in the normally sterile blood. Septic patients are very sick and will always require hospitalization. They will have an IV and get antibiotics intravenously. Death will occur if treatment is withheld.

Chapter 14

Special issues associated with dementia

Advanced Directives

Regulations and laws vary relative to pre-arranged directives for specific medical treatments or continued life support after one has become too confused to make that decision. It is probably a good idea for everyone to address this issue early as we never know if there might be a catastrophic event where this decision might come into play. Leaving a family or spouse to make such a choice is stressful and often leads to conflict. Certainly anyone with early dementia should have some legal statement on file addressing how to proceed in the terminal phases of life.

This should also include direction about resuscitation. Resuscitation is somewhat different than other life support or treatment issues in that it addresses what to do in the event of an emergency where there may be a sudden loss of life. The question then becomes – should there be an aggressive response including CPR or cardiopulmonary resuscitation. CPR is of course an important immediate response to an event where loss of life seems imminent. Most are not aware however that the survival rate after CPR is low, somewhere around five percent. Many who do survive suffer permanent brain injury from time spent without oxygen to the brain. Additionally, the process of applying repeated pressure to the chest is traumatic and ribs can be broken. Understanding the details of CPR will often make the elderly think twice about opting for this procedure. Advanced directive can easily be written by consulting an attorney familiar with family or elder issues.

Driving

We spend most of our life at an age where we can drive. During that period nearly all of us have a driver's license. This is not just a license to drive and have independent transportation but is often our primary source identification. Our driver's license is in effect a symbol of who we are for most of our adult lives. Not surprisingly, the thought of losing one's license can be terrifying and is often met with resistance. Many older people may still qualify for a driver's license but have a diminished ability to drive. Many with dementia who would no longer qualify for a license continue to drive anyway.

As we get older our neurologic system begins to fade. Our reaction time is diminished and our judgment is not as crisp. There are other physical issues such as poor vision and arthritis that may add to the difficulty of managing a car. It should be no surprise then that the added detriment of the memory impairment and diminished orientation make driving a disaster in the making.

The age group with the most non-alcohol related road fatalities are those 65 and older. Many of those are female passengers riding in the right front seat. The male driver makes a left turn in front of oncoming traffic and they are "t-boned". The left turn is a maneuver that exploits all of the dangers of an elderly demented driver. The arthritis makes the quick movements required to accomplish the turn before the on coming car arrives harder. The poor vision makes it difficult to judge how far away the oncoming care is. The slow reaction time slows the initiation of the turn. Finally, any dementia and all of the related anxious confusion of the moment diminishes the driver's capacity to make a snap decision and find a safe way out of the danger.

Families will often approach the doctor and ask for advice or even make a request to have the patient terminated from driving. They even may ask the doctor to tell the dementia patient that he or she cannot drive any more. Obviously this can get complicated. While it is true that most people with dementia should not drive, the process of getting there may require a great deal of energy and creativity. One way to make things easier is to anticipate the problem and make a process out of it. Start early and ease into the change. Generally when a doctor notifies a governmental department of licensing that the patient has dementia they will terminate the license. This step would best occur after a transitional period where the patient has become accustomed to and provided with other modes of transportation. Ample time must be allowed to work through the change emotionally.

The spouse

The spouse is often over looked during the course of treatment of dementia. The hidden story when dementia emerges amidst a relationship, particularly a lengthy one, is the slow and agonizing separation. Dementia carries with it all the stress of a traumatic divorce with the added humility and devastation of one partner often not being a willing or able participant any longer.

Obviously, relationships differ in quality and the loss of a partner may have different meanings. What seems unique about dementia is the slow nature of the separation. Early on, there may well be considerable opportunity for denial on a spouse's part as the symptoms are often subtle. Without realizing it, one can easily enable the mentally debilitated partner by helping out a little here and there or changing the life style to a simpler one. Such a response will almost certainly occur if there is secondary gain for the healthy spouse. This may be in delaying the acquisition of dreaded new responsibilities such as financial management or family decision-making. On a deeper level it may mean delaying the feelings of loss or the fear of being alone in the world after a lifetime of partnership.

Sooner or later it will become necessary for the spouse to face the diagnosis of dementia and make some hard decisions about living arrangements or even long-term care. A visit to a long-term care attorney or advisor is often helpful for a couple of reasons. First, in the US, one must have a financial plan to pay for dementia care. In many cases this will involve the ultimate goal of making the demented spouse eligible for Medicaid. This is because Medicaid will often pay for long term care however that requires that the patient not have much in terms of other available resources. This leads to the second reason for the financial advice - to protect the healthy spouse's retirement so it is not all lost in dementia care.

Many spouses are also involved in the medical aspects of care. They may have particular thoughts about what kind of doctor manages the dementia as well as which medications are used. Seeing one's loved one deteriorate can be overwhelming and the spouse may need to seek help for themselves. This may mean an Alzheimer support group or just activities with friends. Formal treatment of anxiety or depression may also be necessary. The bottom line is that spouses should never allow themselves to burn out – not out of guilt, not out of anything. If a nursing home is the best option at the time, do it. No one can give love if they are angry and frustrated.

Sexuality

Sexuality is a basic part of our lives. While things do eventually slow down, sex is not necessarily over as we age. This is true as well for those stricken with dementia. There is commonly a diminution of sexual behavior in dementia however an augmentation or even inappropriate sexual behavior may also occur. For this reason, the subject of sexuality does very much recall the notion of the wandering explorer. While attempting to accept dementia patients for who they are and allow them to be active, sexual behavior may require careful consideration.

In the first place, while difficult to predict, some dementia patients may have a heightened sense of sexual arousal. Additionally, they may become disinhibited, just like with alcohol delirium. They may want it and want it now. The object of sexual desire may be someone mistaken for the spouse or even some other partner out of the past. Or maybe is just doesn't matter who it is.

In any event, some decisions need to be made. Things are easiest if the patient is living with the spouse and the focus of sexual interest is that person. Obviously, things get much more problematic when other people are involved. Sexual advances towards others are generally considered inappropriate however consideration must be given to the nature of what might be a developing and caring relationship with another patient. Part of active wandering and exploring could also include sexual interest towards caregivers. This behavior may promote socialization or mood stabilization and be an important aspect of the patient's day. For this reason it is crucial that caregivers be trained in the proper management and response to such behavior.

A classic problem that occurs is a female caregiver and a confused male patient. Not realizing she has played a role in the development of the problem, she may have kissed him on the cheek from time to time, called him honey, or even shared with him some of her own personal saga. The patient, lonely and disinhibited, enjoys her company. It doesn't take long before he crosses the line with a comment or a touch. The caregiver suddenly finds herself feeling uncomfortable or even angry. This prompts a report of the event and an intervention ensues. Unfortunately the intervention may mean a serious medication change, hospitalization or even dismissal from the facility. There are of course cases where caregivers are the victims of unprovoked advances where a serious and immediate intervention needs to be made.

Similar scenarios may unfold in assisted living or skilled nursing facilities with other dementia patients. This may range from a subtle attraction and companionship to frank sexual assault. Obviously, as with caregiver issues, different situations require different management. There is one situation that may occur between patients in a facility that is not likely to happen with a caregiver. From time to time, one sees a relationship develop between two confused patients. It may start very subtly as a friendship or companionship and later become something more. The participants often have similar levels of confusion following an old rule that is true for all of us where like quantities of psychopathology tend to attract one another. Anything other than that would prompt a discussion about how able the participants are to acknowledge and understand what they are doing. This is obviously an ethically charged issue that will involve facility administrative and clinical staff as well as family and perhaps even a spouse. In the end, some patients are actually allowed a space and time to consummate their desire.

An interesting feature we have noticed with patients over the years has to do with sexual orientation. It has been our experience that patients who are known to be homosexual remain so until the end. They can forget how to brush their teeth or even eat. They can no longer remember when to empty their bowels or when it is appropriate to laugh or cry. But they will still be gay. It does seem to support the contention that sexual orientation is an inherent aspect of ourselves we are born with rather than a learned behavior.

The following are some basic guidelines to help deal with sexual behavior in dementia patients:

1. As with any of us, sexual behavior in a dementia may or may not be pathologic.

2. Understand what, if any, provoking issues may be occurring on the part of staff or other patients and limit them.

3. Non-spousal caregivers should never: encourage sexual behavior, behave sexually in the presence of patients, or use provocative language.

4. All intimacy between caregivers and patients should be carefully thought through. This should include but not be limited to kissing, hugging, unusual amounts of one on one time together and the sharing of personal information.

5. Caregivers should never allow themselves to get in harms way. Avoid any situation that may lead to physical entrapment. Physical caregiving should be done with partners in all questionable cases.

6. Should it be determined that further intervention is required, attempt to explain to the patient what the concerns are in a non-threatening manner.

7. Redirect the patient away from any situation that may escalate into the problematic behavior while encouraging neutral socialization.

8. Assess the patient medically for delirium or medication effects. Antidepressants may cause hypersexual behavior.

9. If the behavior is persisting and clearly pathologic, consider a psychiatric consultation to address the need for a mood stabilizer or antipsychotic. Sedative hypnotics and alcohol should be avoided.

10. Some sexual behavior between patients may be normal and allowed but only after careful consideration by the families and professionals.

Violence

Unfortunately, violence is commonplace in the management of dementia. Disinhibition, mood instability, confusion and psychosis are some of the common causes of this phenomenon. Additionally there is the depression and aggravation associated with all the medical, social and financial issues that the demented elderly are confronted with. This makes for an explosive mix that is truly unique. At no other time in life are we confronted with more stress that we are unable to cope with. The result may range from the sudden onset of verbal or physical outbursts that is predictable and perhaps associated with caregiving to an unprovoked attack upon another patient or caregiver that is later found to be well calculated. Fortunately, the later is not common as it may result in serious injury or death. That is not to underplay the more common situational violence. Either staff or caregivers may be seriously injured at any time however much can be accomplished in identifying and preventing this form of attack.

By far the bulk of aggressive behavior occurs during caregiving. Any change in tone or manner should be considered to possibly be a threatening posture. Usually, it is quite obvious that the patient is irritated and not happy with something that may be going on. Do not push it. You will be injured. An appropriate response is to terminate the current event or situation and return to something more routine and neutral. That previous situation or activity should not be entered into again until help is available. A clear plan of physical escape should always be thought through whenever working one on one with a patient with dementia.

Sundowning

Sundowning is a peculiar phenomenon seen in dementia where patients will become more confused and thus psychiatrically symptomatic in the afternoon and evening hours. It will often begin in the early afternoon just after lunch and reach a peak in the early evening. Planning for this with more complex tasks such as doctor visits in the morning is always a good idea. Napping in the afternoon may be helpful however there is commonly nothing that can prevent some sundowning. Often medications that are meant to calm or help with symptoms such as psychosis will be prescribed in the early afternoon and evening rather than the morning.

Personalities

Our personality is the core of who we are. It is the complex mix of the hard neurologic wiring we were born with and the knee jerk emotional reactions we have developed through our early life experiences. The former is a powerful fact of inheritance and is not well understood. No one knows why, of two siblings raised similarly, that one might be obsessive and the other narcissistic. Certainly the early dynamics in the relationships we have with our parents can be better understood and traceable. Child abuse of any kind will always have a negative impact on the personality.

As a person gets older the personality does not go away. While virtually anything can happen with dementia, there is a general trend for problem personalities to become more expansive and even problematic. An obsessive type may well become a hoarder, a pessimist a depressive, and a narcissist -

paranoid. I wish I could say that all calm and even keel people facing dementia would remain so but we know that is not always the case. It is not clear whether or not new or problematic features of a person dealing with dementia are due to some previously hidden aspect of themselves or just a different or new part of the brain that is being challenged. I have had suspected both from time to time.

Chapter 15

Environmental options

Not enough can be said about the importance of the living environment in the management of dementia. Even if the most we can expect to achieve is a pleasantly confused wandering explorer, the living situation will have as much of an impact as anything else in accomplishing and maintaining that goal. Demented or not, our home is our space where we can just be. When we are "in" we are at home. When we are "out" we are not at home. It's where our stuff is. It's where people come to see us if we want and it's where we retreat to when we want to avoid seeing people. It might be where we grew up. It might be where we had a relationship or raised kids. Whatever it is, our living situation is something that is so familiar to us that it is in itself therapeutic, especially if we are confused.

Beyond that and environment can be adapted in many ways to provide for structure, for safety, for accessibility, and for a zillion other aspects of life that one might think of to provide for living and for comfort. In this chapter we will explore some of the different living situations relative to dementia. We'll keep in mind that structure and social interaction are generally important contributors to the psychological welfare of people with dementia. It must also be stated that at the writing of this book the American (and likely other countries involved with WWII) baby boomers are just on the cusp of being of age to get dementia. My prediction is that the industry of long term care is about to explode. Let's look at the environmental options.

Home

Home is where the heart is, right? Well, maybe. Most people prefer to stay in a private home, whether a house or an apartment, as long as possible. This is generally true of dementia patients and their families as well. In fact, most with dementia in the US are living at a private home. After all, particularly in the early stages of memory loss, there is little reason not to. A familiar environment that, if adapted a little for safety or accessibility, is perfect. Home is usually cheap too when compared to other living situations. Many patients are fortunate enough to live out their lives at home. But for others comes a time where things might go better outside the home.

If the private home does eventually become less attractive as an option, the reasons might be either: an increased need for medical care or behaviors. The former is not necessarily a dementia related issue and could happen to anyone who is older. The second, the behaviors, are very much a product dementia.

I would divide the potential home behavior problems into two groups. The first is the potential isolation of home. What used to be a place to retreat on a bad day and regroup can become a place for continuous refuge from the world. What if every day is bad? This happens in many cases of dementia as anxieties about memory problems and being "found out" in social situations evolve. This is often the beginning of a larger problem. Social isolation will cause the anxiety and depression to worsen to the point that an intervention of some kind may be necessary. If not, nutrition and basic needs usually suffer will and culminate in medical consequences. Furthermore, the lack of reality testing in the world outside the house may lead to paranoia and psychosis.

And then, someone with more advanced dementia is going to wander. This often happens at odd hours. They may have mood swings with agitation. They may need coaxing to take meds, to bathe or to eat. Clearly then, a point is reached where "home alone" is no longer an option. Eventually, continuous nursing care or observation is required. This must either be brought in or provided by the family. Most families cannot provide nursing care nor can they be available night after night to prevent wandering. This generally leads to burn out.

The classic situation we have seen at out clinic are the dedicated spouses who vowed never to put their loved one into a nursing home and are running themselves into the ground. In some cases it is the healthy spouse's fear of being alone after sixty years of partnership that prevents exploration of better options. In others it is commitment. In still others it is guilt. Once able to look at the options, the expense of bringing help into the home will make most reconsider other alternatives. One thing that generally must occur outside the home is the visit to the doctor as few of us make house calls anymore.

Assisted Living

In the US, assisted living generally is a means of retaining some degree of independence and yet having varying degrees of assistance at hand. Typically, assisted living is appropriate for early to middle stages of dementia although more and more do advanced care as well. Individuals and couples will likely have their own room that may have a variety of accessories depending on the facility. Meals are usually provided in a central dining area with other services such as light nursing care, medications, and cleaning available. Another attractive feature is that help is always just seconds away. Because the facility is staffed twenty four hours a day, wandering issues are easily dealt with. Assisted living is not cheap. Costs usually range from $4000 to $8000 per month.

The higher end facilities are usually private pay and do not accept Medicaid. While there is some degree of governmental regulation of assisted living it is not nearly as intense as that for skilled nursing facilities.

Adult Family Homes

Adult family homes often care for patients with similar levels of impairment to assisted living. They are commonly run by a person with some history in heath care who has a large home and makes a business out of caring for four or six people. Obviously this option provides a more intimate setting that can be very attractive to many families. Many who do well in this setting are in need of social attention and tend to get lost in the more crowded facilities. Like assisted living there is a great deal of care provided with considerable independence as well.

Costs tend to be cheaper than assisted living and Medicaid acceptance is the rule. Regulatory levels are similar to that of assisted living.

Skilled Nursing facilities

Skilled nursing facilities (SNFs) are what used to be known as nursing homes in the US. The name change would suggest an increased level of sophistication and this is generally the case. There are a few reasons for this. In the first place, changes in the insurance reimbursement system have forced much shorter hospitalizations for many medical problems. There then arose a need for a place for continued care between the hospital and home. Also, the development of the art and science of long term care has led to a much different role in skilled nursing than was the case even fifteen years ago. This is very much a function of the fact that there are more old people and they are living longer.

While there are still many general care facilities one of the most noticeable changes has been a specialization. Many facilities are now called rehab centers, focusing on post hospitalization nursing care. Another large area of specialization has been in dementia. Most facilities, regardless of specialization, are aware of the need to have expertise in the management of dementia because of its prevalence in long term care.

SNFs are highly regulated by the government. Some actually ask for accreditation on the level of hospitals and use that fact to gain the confidence of the public. Traditionally nursing homes were seen as dangerous warehouses. This can no longer be the case as even the idle care of a patient nowadays is considered dangerous neglect. Such care would certainly lead to a citation and possible further action.

In skilled nursing facilities, patients have hospital like rooms. They may or may not share a room. The intensity of nursing staff and their qualifications is generally a step up from assisted living. All patients have a physician who must see the patient at regular intervals there at the facility.

Without question, many skilled nursing facilities are not the most pleasant places to visit. They are however, necessary and will be playing an ever more important role in healthcare. These facilities are often the ultimate place to care for people in the later stages of dementia although it must be said that some assisted livings and adult family homes are quite capable of seeing the disease through to completion. Families often change their view of such facilities after they are forced to send a member to a skilled nursing facility only to find the care is good and far beyond whet could have been accomplished elsewhere.

In the US, skilled nursing facilities are often at the mercy of sudden visits from the government. The cost of maintaining currency with all the regulatory requirements as well as offering sometimes advanced medical capabilities is great. This often translates to higher cost to the patient. Generally families are facing $5000 to $8000 per month in skilled nursing. Medicare will cover medical problems for ninety days. Sadly, dementia is not considered a medical problem that warrants such coverage. Long term care insurance will pay but most don't have it. Families are then faced with either paying privately or finding some way to get the patient on Medicaid. This is a dance for which an elder law attorney or financial planner is like gold.

Dementia units

Otherwise known as Alzheimer care facilities, they are what they say - facilities that specialize in the long term management dementia and its peculiar issues. Behavioral challenges are one of the primary missions of such facilities. As you are now aware these behaviors range from wandering and exploring to agitation Violence and inappropriate sexual activity are commonplace.

Some dementia facilities are assisted living while others are skilled nursing at their core. The former included some of the most beautiful, creative and well run facilities available. The latter usually implies an added level of in-house consultation and service intensity as well as certainty of maximum regulation by the state. All of these facilities are secured at some point from the inside. The cost of dementia care at the higher end facilities is very expensive. Medicaid will not be accepted at most.

Chapter 16

Behavioral management

Behavioral management in dementia care is often considered to be that care that does not involve the use of medication. The reality is that it is most commonly used in tandem with medication. If, however, there is a way of minimizing medication then I am all for it. A close proximity of personal versed in such techniques is definitively one of those ways. This area can be divided into three basic areas: environmental considerations, specific triggers of stress, and psychological techniques.

Environment Considerations

It is well documented that older patients, particularly those with dementia, may have a powerful therapeutic response to the environment. An example of this is the difficulty researchers have had in measuring the efficacy of antidepressants in the elderly. This is because the enrollment and initial evaluation of depressed elderly patients in the research projects is such a powerful antidepressant in itself that depression significantly resolves before a drug is even started. In these cases social stimulation and the mere interest of others is introduced into the lives of some very lonely and under stimulated individuals. The response is dramatic.

The long-term care industry has put this phenomenon to use by intentionally integrating socially appealing and stimulating atmospheres into assisted living and skilled nursing facilities. While often dismissed by families as a viable long-term option, long-term care providers realize that many patients are neglected and under stimulated at home. Such patients are often depressed and generally more anxious and agitated than those who are in more social environments.

That is not to say that being at home when older or demented is wrong, but consider some facts. Physically, the elderly and confused people are more prone to falls and less able to provide care for themselves. Why then wouldn't it also be true that those same people would require more assistance from an emotional point of view? We who may not be elderly or confused take for granted the various options we have to escape our anxieties. We can go out to a movie or dinner, chat on line, or undertake any number of intellectual pursuits. Ever see a couple go out to dinner together and then each pull out a separate book or magazine to read? True, they may be enjoying the dinner and the reading, but they are more than likely unaware of the anxiety and depression relief they are attaining.

If you think about it, depression and anxiety relief are the reason behind why we do many activities. The relief feels good, sometimes physically and almost always mentally. Unfortunately, the elderly and certainly those with confusion have fewer options in this regard. They are often left to feel their depression and anxieties unabated by activity.

Identification of Specific Triggers

Any of us can become a psychiatric patient with the right environmental trigger. It may be something specific for us as individuals such as the sudden appearance of someone or something out of the past that is associated with a traumatic experience or something more collective that would upset anyone such as a severe illness, loss or other catastrophe. We have discussed how those who are elderly or demented are more vulnerable to delirium due to metabolic changes in their bodies. Similarly, changes in the environment can be more mentally upsetting and symptomatic for this group as well.

To someone with dementia a room change in a nursing home could have the same impact that a stressful experience like selling a home or moving away might have on a younger person. Given this sensitivity of the elderly, it is important that caregivers explore for environmental change issues in the face of any new mental status change, especially in those who have dementia. Environmental triggers are generally easily identifiable, easy to solve, and a way of avoiding more complex solutions such as medication or a hospitalization.

Psychological techniques

Some psychiatric events will happen in those with dementia regardless of a socially stimulating environment and may not always be associated with any identifiable emotional trigger. Still, the avoidance of medication should be attempted due to the sensitivities the elderly and demented have. As mentioned previously, an exploration of medical causes of behavioral changes should always be pursued first. The medical workup is commonly negative however. Consider then that delirium is ruled out. There are no specific triggers identified and the environment is safe and stimulating. When then should medication be entertained? The answer is probably immediately if there is a threat or danger to self or others. If there is time however, a behavioral or psychological approach should be considered first.

Depending upon the nature of the problem and level of confusion this may be something simple like redirecting a very confused person from a problematic situation to one that is less so. Other times the patient may be more cognitively aware and a half hour of talking and trying to work through a problem psychologically may be beneficial. One form of talking that is often employed with those who are confused is called validation. This technique might also be called caregiver acceptance. Most of the crazy and confused thought avenues are accepted and validated as though they were real.

This process avoids conflict with the caregiver and may give a patient a sense of purpose and being normal. Obviously a point may come where such avenues are distressing or dangerous and limits may need to be set with redirection to another place, either physically or psychologically employed. One obvious instance of a difficult situation where validation is not going to work is paranoia. "You want me dead. You want all I have". You do not have to be a dementia expert to see that agreeing with this proposition is not a good idea.

In practice then, things like paranoia happen and nothing seems to work the way it might in some book or chapter on behavior techniques. Even if medications are started, behavioral techniques or at least a provision for an environment that is calming, structured and yet socially stimulating will generally be of benefit. The fact of the matter is that the appropriate use of environmental, psychological and pharmacologic interventions is generally considered to be a sound approach to any neurologic or psychiatric problem.

Chapter 17

Dementia and medication

Pharmacology is the science of medication. In particular, neuropharmacology and psychopharmacology are the specific disciplines involved in the medication management of dementia. Let's be clear from the start. While there is a great deal of excitement and interest in this area by many groups, there is currently no known medication that cures dementia.

Only acetylcholinesterase inhibitors and a NMDA antagonist known as memantine have been found consistently to temporarily improve the symptoms of or more importantly delay the progression of dementia. There are no vitamins, herbs or other medical remedies that have been demonstrated in randomized double blind controlled studies (the gold standard of research) to consistently effect dementia. There are many who would argue with this point and I say to them – show me the study. Some researchers at universities are conducting cutting edge research and may indeed have something to offer in clinical studies of new products that we may hear about soon. But beware. There are also many fanatics out there. They know you want to help your loved one. They also know many families will often do anything. It's like cancer but with even less options. Generally, you will get nothing for your money and be left with more heartache, and frustration.

I have already expressed my criticism of the pharmaceutical industry and the academic community for what I believe is an over emphasis on Alzheimer's disease. To be clear, I do not feel there is less dementia than they do not do nor do I think that Alzheimer's disease does not exist. I just think there is more of a blood vessel and normal aging component that has been left out of the equation in the service of putting the emphasis on aspects of dementia that are more consistent with the actions of the medications they are selling. That said, and in full disclosure, I do support the use of these medications for reasons I will describe. Over the past ten years I have been a paid speaker for some of the pharmaceutical companies and have helped them market their medications for dementia. I have not been silent about my concerns, however, during conversations with the company representatives and during my presentations when allowed. Two companies continue to offer me a speaking contract which I accept.

There are two general groups of medications used in the treatment of dementia. The first are medications actually approved by the Food and Drug Administration (FDA) for an indication to treat dementia. As mentioned above these are acetylcholinesterase inhibitors and the NMDA antagonist called memantine.

The other group is the psychiatric medications. They are used to manage many of the symptoms of the disease as it progresses. As previously mentioned psychiatric symptoms are very common in dementia. Few patients will progress through the course of the disease without receiving some psychiatric medication. These medications are commonly divided into four major groups: the antipsychotics, the anxiolytics (anti-anxiety medications), the anti-depressants and the mood stabilizers. We shall discuss in detail all the different classes of medication used in treating dementia. Using some examples, we'll take a practical look at the risks and benefits of each.

Neuropsychiatric Medication in General

Most psychiatric medications work by effecting the actions of specific chemicals in the brain. These chemicals are called neurotransmitters. Neurotransmitters work to bridge the gap, called the synapse, between the neurons (nerve cells). Let's see how it all works. A message or nerve impulse travels electrically down the long wire like body of the nerve cell. The message could be for any number of actions: to move a foot, to feel a feeling, to bring a memory into awareness. There are always at least two nerve cells involved (usually thousands or millions) in any action and therefore the electrical impulse must be passed from at least one nerve cell to another. The electrical impulse cannot arc across the space between the cells (the synapse) as one might imagine. Rather, it is transformed into a chemical message at the terminal end of one nerve cell, carried across the synapse in the form of a neurotransmitter, and received by a receptor on the next nerve cell only to be switched back to an electrical message and carried away.

As mentioned, most psychiatric medications work by effecting the actions of neurotransmitters and it is in or near the synapse where most neurotransmitters can be found. The specific effect of each medication is different. It may change the amount of neurotransmitter released, affect its breakdown or re-uptake from the synapse back into the cell, modulate or block the receptor or have any number of ways to change the action of the neurotransmitter. The net effect is a modification of brain activity. Okay, let's take a look at the specific medications.

Cholinesterase Inhibitors

The cholinesterase inhibitors were the first class of drugs to be approved for the treatment of dementia. It all began with Tacrine in the early 1990s followed by Aricept in the mid 90s. Exelon arrived in 1997 and then finally there came Reminyl in early 2000. The specific FDA indication for all four medications has been the treatment of mild to moderate Alzheimer type dementia with three exceptions: Aricept is approved for mild, moderate and advanced disease and

Exelon is approved for Parkinson dementia as well as Alzheimer's disease. Namenda is approved for moderate to severe Alzheimer dementia.

Acetylcholine is a major chemical (neurotransmitter) in our nervous system. It is involved with thinking, memory and many other brain and nerve functions. In particular acetylcholine plays a vital role with short-term memory in an area of the brain known as the hippocampus. Medications that are "cholinergic" enhance the acetylcholine system. Those that are anti-cholinergic work against it.

Research has determined there to be a deterioration of the brain's acetylcholine and the cholinergic system in Alzheimer's disease. Cholinesterase inhibitors enhance the cholinergic system in the brain by increasing the levels of acetylcholine. This is accomplished by neutralizing acetylcholinesterase, the enzyme that breaks down acetylcholine - thus the name "cholinesterase inhibitor".

The studies done on these medications have clearly demonstrated the ability to delay the progression of some cognitive symptoms of Alzheimer's disease. By this we mean a delay in the deterioration of short-term memory, orientation and other basic thinking functions. As one might imagine, this may have secondary beneficial effects on other measures such as psychosis, anxiety and depression. Indeed such effects have been documented in studies also demonstrating a reduction in caregiver burden and over-all cost of care.

This would be a good point to remind ourselves that anticholinergic medications, those that work against acetylcholine, are potential confusion enhancers. While there is no data they cause dementia, they certainly may cause delirium and can work against the action of the cholinesterase inhibitors.

The anticholinergic effect is a common property found in many medications:

Lasix
Digoxin
Coumadin
Codeine
Detrol
Benadryl
Zantac
Theophylline
Hydrochlorothiazide
Nifedipine
Captopril
Thorazine
Mellaril
Elavil
Tofranil
Desipramine
Sinequan
Paxil
Zyprexa
Clozaril

Note that many of the older antidepressants (Tofranil, Sinequan, and Elavil) and antipsychotics (Mellaril, Thorazine) have this property. Resolving this has been part of the improvement with the newer generation of psychiatric medications although even some newer ones have some anticholinergic activity (Paxil, Zyprexa). While the classic anticholinergic side effects are dry mouth, blurred vision and constipation; delirium with confusion and visual hallucinations can easily occur. Obviously, some such medications may be necessary but one must keep in mind that the effect can be cumulative and a general trend to limit such medications should always be a part of dementia management.

As a rule the cholinesterase inhibitors should be taken with food to avoid the sudden surge of cholinergic activity responsible for the most common side effects – nausea and vomiting. Increasing the doses slowly towards the therapeutic dose is also important to avoid such side effects. Let's look at each medication specifically.

Tacrine

This was the first of the cholinesterase inhibitors to be approved for the treatment of mild to moderate Alzheimer dementia. While still available, this medication has lost favor in the US due to side effects related to the liver.

Aricept (donepezil)

The ease of once a day dosing and a starting dose being a potentially therapeutic one has helped to make this medication popular. Doses begin at 5mg daily and should be increased to 10mg after 2 months. The mechanism of action of Aricept is by sole inhibition of acetyl cholinesterase. Aricept is generally well tolerated. Problematic side effects are nausea, vomiting or diarrhea. Aricept is metabolized through the liver and its enzymes. Potential drug-drug interactions exist but this is generally not a problem.

Exelon (rivastigmine)

This medication is an inhibitor of both acetyl and butyrylcholinesterase. While the exact role of butyrylcholinesterase remains unclear, its levels are raised in the short-term memory part of the brain in Alzheimer dementia. This second action has been marketed as the dual edged sword for this medication. This is a twice a day medication that is very potent and rapidly absorbed. Exelon must be given with food with the dose not increased sooner than once every two months to avoid the usual side effects of nausea and vomiting. Dosing starts at 1.5mg twice daily with an increase to 3mg twice daily after two months, then 4.5mg twice daily after 4 months and a final dose of 6mg twice a day after 6 months. Therapeutic benefit may be seen at the lower doses although benefit clearly has a linear relationship to dose. Exelon is metabolized and excreted through the kidney making for minimal drug-drug interactions.

Because of side effects with the oral medication, Exelon is now available as a 24 hour daily patch. This route of administration is much better tolerated. It is available as a 4.6mg patch for one month then maintenance on a 9.5mg patch.

Razadyne (galantamine)

Razadyne used to be called Reminyl. It is an acetyl cholinesterase inhibitor with receptor modulation capacity as well. This means that Razadyne can additionally increase acetylcholine activity through an entirely different manner. Razadyne is metabolized and excreted through both the liver and kidney. It must be given twice a day and the dose must be increased from the initial starting dose of 4mg twice a day to 8mg twice daily, 12mg twice daily and finally 16mg twice daily. Dose increases should be spaced by 2 months and Razadyne should be given with food to avoid the nausea and vomiting. There is an extended release for available for once daily dosing.

NMDA Inhibitors

NMDA or N-methyl D-aspartate receptors are involved with changes in the voltage potential between the inside and outside of the brain cells. This voltage potential in turn is directly associated with the activation and propagation of nerve impulses. The NMDA receptors therefore are closely associated with vital brain activities including thinking and memory. Glutamate is a neurotransmitter that attaches to NMDA receptors and causes electrical excitation of nerve cells. The glutamate system has been found to function in a hyperactive and therefore toxic manner in Alzheimer dementia. By blocking the glutamate stimulation of the NMDA receptor, thus better regulating nerve cell activity, the dementia process can be slowed and cognitive symptoms improved.

Namenda (memantine) is a NMDA inhibitor that has been used for dementia in Europe for many years. This medication got approval by the FDA for the treatment of moderate to severe dementia in the US in early 2004. This and Aricept are currently the only medications approved for use in the more advanced cases although all the cholinesterase inhibitors have been shown to limit caregiver burden and the use of psychiatric medication in advanced dementia.

In fact, a combination of memantine with a cholinesterase inhibitor may be the most prudent treatment regardless of the stage. This was suggested by some study trials with the combination of Aricept with memantine showing better efficacy than Aricept or memantine alone and little drug-drug interaction problems. Others have found that Razadyne and Exelon seem to work well with memantine also.

Namenda, alone or in combination, is generally well tolerated however it is recommended that the medication dose be increased from 5mg daily over four weeks to a final dose of 20mg a day. The cost of Namenda is comparable to the cholinesterase inhibitors making combination therapy about $300 monthly. Remember that studies have shown that both cholinesterase inhibitors and NMDA inhibitors in combination or alone may cut the cost of caregivers and\or medication thus making them financially viable. This result, unfortunately, cannot be guaranteed.

It should be noted that, in the US, the current standard of care is that all cases of Alzheimer dementia should be given a trial on one of these mediations. While none of them have clearly been shown to outperform the others, combined therapy between memantine and one of the three cholinesterase inhibitors is generally considered optimal even in the early stages of the illness. Life will not be prolonged but one can expect a relative delay of symptom progression over a two to three year period if the drug is started early. The later the start the less robust the result in general although an occasional later stage patient may benefit significantly.

Anti-psychotics

The anti-psychotics are a class of medications that carry a controversy very much paralleling problem they treat. Few things are more mysterious and frightening to the general population than psychosis. This is partially because of the sometimes-bizarre nature of this phenomenon but perhaps more so because of the unconscious potential for any of us to become psychotic. Studies have shown that the ultimate anxiety in human beings seems to relate to a sense of mental annihilation or losing ones mind. It is of no surprise then that those who require anti-psychotic medication are often agitated, anxious, or depressed. To many, the anti-psychotics conger up images of crazed schizophrenics being injected and tied down by men in white coats in the back wards of state hospitals. The reality is that these medications helped to prevent such scenes.

Also known as neuroleptics, the antipsychotics were originally classed as major tranquilizers. This classification separated them from the minor tranquilizers or sedative hypnotics of which Valium is the classic. Thorazine (chlorpromazine), the first ant-psychotic, was discovered to be a useful medication for psychosis in the early 1950s and was soon followed by Haldol (haloperidol). Up until the arrival of these two medications those with psychotic conditions were not uncommonly treated with lobotomies, insulin shock therapy, and long-term hospitalization. The fact is that antipsychotic medication has advanced the treatment of chronic mental illness to the point where the largest hospitals in the human history, the American state mental institutions (some with 30,000 plus beds is some cases), have dramatically dwindled in size.

While the newer medications are more complex, antipsychotics in general function in lowering symptoms of psychosis by blocking one of the crucial neurotransmitters involved in our thinking. This natural brain chemical is called dopamine. Without it we are left with a blank expression and a paucity of thought, not unlike people with Parkinson's disease (PD), an illness of dopamine depletion. Unfortunately, Parkinsonism, a name for a syndrome that looks like PD, has been a side effect of antipsychotics. This has led to a sense that these medications may cause a "zombification" of the patient. And such a result truly may be achieved with high enough doses of any antipsychotic. For this reason doctors are trained to understand medication side effects and use them judiciously.

Dementia is an illness where psychosis is commonplace. Hallucinations may occur and delusions can take the form of paranoid ideas or mistaken identity. The thought process may be so disturbed that it is expressed verbally as a word salad. These disturbances of perception, thought content and thought process are the typical ingredients of psychosis. In the case of dementia one might liken the pathologic event to a dashboard fire in a car whereby the overheated wires melt together fusing the circuits of thought. It is as though there is a smoke clouding the understanding and the fire of roaring and bizarre ideas. What better thing to do to ameliorate the situation than to simply lower the voltage. A good result might be to cut down as much of the fire and smoke as possible while preserving what instruments and gauges that one can. Voltage in the thinking brain is dopamine.

The good news about antipsychotics and dementia is that very low doses can be used to accomplish a lot. This single factor makes these medications tremendously more useful because the lower doses cause fewer side effects. The other side of the argument is that the fragile dementia patient could never tolerate the higher doses anyway.

Equally important, psychotic dementia patients are often anxious, depressed, or emotionally unstable. Such patients are commonly medicated with three four or five different medications to treat all these different problems. The medications mix and the side effects mount. Before long the patient is lethargic and delirious. Quite often several psychiatric concerns can be treated solely with a very low dose of an antipsychotic. Not only are they indicated for mood disorders but by lowering the "voltage" enough to take the psychotic edge off, the depression and anxiety may lift as well. The antipsychotics, therefore, are one of the most important classes of medications in one's armamentarium during the course of management of psychiatric aspects of dementia. Sadly, families and many general practitioners are often misinformed and uncomfortable with this group of medications and will opt to stay away from them until "later on".

In certain cases, even low doses of anti-psychotic medication may overmedicate a patient. As the disease evolves, the patient may become more vulnerable to side effects and can become overmedicated with doses that were once successfully managing a problem. The most common side effects of the antipsychotics are due generally to the dopamine blockade and in particular in a part of the brain known as the basal ganglia. The tremor, flat gaze, rigid muscle tone seen in Parkinson's patients may be seen in non-Parkinson patients who are not tolerating the medication. These side effects are known as EPS or extrapyramidal side effects. Other problems can be falls or lethargy but these side effects must be put into perspective. Lethargy at night may be a good thing. And, while falls are never a good result, there is data to suggest that antipsychotics may prevent falls in certain dosages. This is because psychosis and agitation are in themselves risk factors for falls.

It should be noted that all antipsychotics will lower the seizure threshold thus making it more likely to have a seizure in someone with a risk such as a history of seizures, a stroke or a tumor. Those who are already on medications for seizures can be given antipsychotic safely; however, I will usually try a mood stabilizer such as Depakote first in a high risk patient. Let's, look at some of the advantages and disadvantages of the different antipsychotic medications.

Typical (older) anti-psychotics

Death directly associated with anti-psychotics is a rare event. When it does occur it is generally seen in a syndrome known as NMS or neuroleptic malignant syndrome. NMS may be seen with all anti-psychotic medication but it is much more commonly associated with the older medications. Dopamine affects several vital areas of the brain including the thermoregulatory center of the hypothalamus. On occasion, a crisis may occur where patients develop a rapidly progressing fever in association with tremor, rigidity, and hypertension. NMS is a medical emergency that requires immediate treatment, generally in the ICU. Management includes discontinuation of the anti-psychotic medication, intravenous hydration, and not uncommonly treatment with Bromocriptine, a medication known to be a dopamine agonist (increase dopamine).

With the use of anti-psychotic medication one also runs the risk of having to deal with a potentially permanent movement disorder known as Tardive Dyskinesia or TD. TD is the result of chronic dopamine blockade. In this case the receptors on the neurons that dopamine is normally transmitted to have been depleted of dopamine by virtue of the medication for so long that they grow large and hypertrophic searching for more. Upon withdrawal from the medication then, one can suddenly have a surge of dopamine (because the blockade is gone) landing upon the overgrown receptors. The result is a dyskinesia or irregular movements often initially involving the mouth but eventually the neck and trunk as well. TD can be very debilitating and, sadly, may be permanent.

TD is a primary reason for using the newer or atypical anti-psychotic medications, as the risk of developing this movement disorder is much less and in fact rare with them. Virtually all people, on the other hand who have chronically been on the older antipsychotic medications will have some degree of TD. Additionally, the elderly are much more prone to the development of TD than younger patients. For example, some studies show that as much as half of elderly patients put on haloperidol will get some degree of TD after one year whereas those on the newer antipsychotics might only develop it rarely if at all. Despite the newer medications being more expensive, this is an obvious reason not to use haloperidol as a first line long term treatment for psychosis in the elderly. On the other hand, TD generally will not develop when used for a short period of time. There may be cases where the best result is obtained with haloperidol after failed trails with the newer medications. Considering the relative short life span of some demented patients, it may well be the medication of choice in some cases.

Haldol (haloperidol) is really the only older antipsychotic medication that still has a use in the elderly. The only exception would be chronically mentally ill patients who have done well on one of the other medications over the years and it just doesn't make sense to make a change. In many ways haloperidol is the original Risperdal, now arguably the most popular antipsychotic worldwide. They were both discovered by the same person (Paul Janssen) and have very similar dosing profiles in the elderly (0.5 – 2.0mg once or twice a day). Both are powerful dopamine blockers and therefore great antipsychotics. The problem with Haldol is that it has more of the extrapyramidal side effects (EPS) associated with it and the risk of TD is there.

One benefit of treating the elderly is that we can often get away with very small doses thus avoiding a lot of the side effects. This is particularly pertinent to medications like haloperidol. Haldol also has a long track record of safe use in virtually all-medical problems except Parkinson's disease and is therefore often seen as a frontline medication for the treatment of agitation in the general hospital, ICU, and emergency department. Haldol is one of the few anti-psychotic medications that can be given intravenously for the acute management of agitation or psychosis in those with only venous access. It is one of the few that can be given intramuscularly.

I will list other older antipsychotics. As stated previously, they have little place in the management of elderly patients.

Thorazine (chlorpromazine)
Stelazine (trifluoperazine)
Navane (thiothixene)
Mellaril (thioridazine)
Prolixin (fluphenazine)
Trilafon (perphenazine)

Atypical (newer) anti-psychotics

The second generation of anti-psychotic medications began with the FDA approval of Clozaril (clozapine) in the mid-1980's. These tend to be more complex molecules however dopamine blockade remains the main avenue for the anti-psychotic result. Another central feature of these newer medications is the blockade of serotonin which seems to "undo" some of the dopamine blockade in the basal ganglia and thus some of the EPS. This remains a problem however, especially in the more potent dopamine blocker, Risperdal.

In the US it is important to realize that atypical anti-psychotics only have the FDA approval or indication for the treatment of schizophrenia and bipolar disorder. Two of them may be used in the treatment of depression as well. None of them have the indication by the FDA for use in psychosis associated with either dementia or delirium. The fact remains however, that there is often little other alternative than to use them. This use is neither unethical nor illegal but it does underscore the need for careful understanding of the risks and benefits of the medications.

When reviewing the literature on the management of psychosis and agitation in the elderly one finds many alternative treatments such as environmental or behavioral approaches. Indeed even other medications such as the anxiolytics (anti-anxiety) medications may be of benefit. In the end, however, there are many cases where acute or intense management is necessary and nothing else will be efficacious. Many studies have shown that anti-psychotics are as or more beneficial than the anxiolytics in the management of agitation in organic brain disease. This is certainly the case with psychosis. Beyond that there is data to indicate the quality of life is often better with rather than without these medications.

Problems have been cited with this group of medications as well. We have discussed NMS, TD, and EPS. While NMS and TD are potential issues with the atypicals they are rare events. EPS is more common especially with a more potent dopamine antagonist like Risperdal.

Adult onset diabetes mellitus or type 2 diabetes has been associated with the atypical anti-psychotics. Each of these medications must carry with it a warning about this condition. The reality is that most studies used to demonstrate efficacy with these medications have been done in schizophrenics, a population with a higher occurrence of type 2 diabetes than is seen in the general population. That said, some studies suggest there still appears to be an unexplained increased incidence of type 2 diabetes in patients on atypical anti-psychotic medication.

The data that I have reviewed shows that, while the risk is small, Clozaril is probably the worst offender followed by Seroquel and Zyprexa. Risperdal appears to have a rate not dissimilar to Haldol, a medication that does not carry the warning.

Another issue that has arisen over recent years is the association of atypical antipsychotics with stroke and death. This has led to a black box warning in the US warning about the use of these medications in dementia. This risk appears to be rooted in some early studies done while attempting to get the indication for use in the elderly. Bear mind that many countries worldwide are very accepting of the atypicals for this purpose. In some of those studies there was a slightly higher but significant risk of stroke and death. The warning was then applied to the entire class of medications across the board.

A couple of points : first of all, many studies have since failed to show the increase risk of serious adverse events including one connected to the National Institute of Mental Health called the Catie-AD study. You will note that the discussion suggests that, despite this, these medications are not useful for the purpose I am suggesting because they were stopped as much as placebo. The fact is that they worked better than placebo in the study but were stopped because of side effects such as Parkinsonism and sedation. Any experienced clinician knows that such side effects are common and the world is not a study where you stop something and quit. You can change the dose or switch to something else.....neither of which went into the equation in this study.

Secondly, we put up with the risks stated in the black box warning and the other side effects noted because having psychosis and agitation is not a benign situation in itself. It too can lead to stroke and death, I feel even more so than these medications. Just like the risks we take with chemotherapy for cancer or open heart surgery for coronary artery disease, the risk benefit ratio must be calculated and considered.

Let's now look at the atypical antipsychotics individually.

Risperdal (risperidone) is one of the most commonly prescribed antipsychotics in the elderly. It is a potent dopamine blocker dosed the same as Haldol (.5mg to 2mg once to twice a day) but generally has less EPS and risk of TD associated with it. Compared to the other atypicals however, this medication probably has more EPS. It is not particularly sedating. Risperdal It is available in an oral solution and a rapidly dissolving tablet called the M-tab. Risperdal is also available in once every two week long lasting injectable form called Risperdal Consta at 25 to 50mg. I have had great success with this medication in patients who will not take medications regularly.

Invega (paliperidone) is a newer antipsychotic that is a relative of Risperdal. I have not used in the elderly. It comes in a very hard pill that cannot be crushed which may make it a difficult one for them. There is, however, a form of this medication called Invega Sustenna that is a once monthly injection. Given the success I've had with the every two week Risperdal Consta, this medication may show great promise.

Zyprexa (olanzapine) is another very commonly prescribed antipsychotic. The dosing is on the order of 2.5mg daily to 10mg daily. It is long lasting and can be dosed once a day. There is a tendency towards less EPS than seen with Risperdal however it may have problems due to its anticholinergic properties noted previously. Zyprexa is available in a rapidly dissolving tab called Zydis and an injectable form for emergencies.

Seroquel (quetiapine) is an antipsychotic of choice for patients with Parkinson's disease or Lewy Body Dementia. This is because there is so little EPS associated with it. Unfortunately it may also be a less potent antipsychotic. Dosing is on the order of 25mg to 600mg daily. Seroquel can be sedating and cause falls. Seroquel is also indicated for the treatment of depression in the US.

Geodon (ziprazidone) does tend to have less EPS side effects. Geodon is available in a short-term injectable form for use in emergencies. It has heart issues which may make for problems in the elderly.

Clozaril (clozapine) is the oldest of the atypical antipsychotics. It came out in the mid 1980's and was initially seen as revolutionary. It has little EPS and is therefore very useful in Parkinson patients. Unfortunately, Clozaril is associated with rare cases of bone marrow shut down. Therefore, one must have a weekly blood draw for blood count monitoring. Clozaril is also associated with seizures, sedation and a drop in blood pressure. Dosing is similar to Seroquel, 25mg to 300mg daily.

Abilify (aripiprazole) is a more recent antipsychotic to come onto the market. This medication has promise as a maintenance medication and has limited side effects. It may be used safely in Lewy body disease and is a once daily drug. It is limited in its use as an initial stabilization medication. Dosing is in the range of 5 to 20 mg in the morning. Activation or even agitation may be initial side effects. Abilify is also indicated for treatment of depression in the US.

Fanapt (iloperidone) is the newest antipsychotic in the US. Is appears to be very well tolerated with minimal Parkinsonism. I have not used it in the elderly. It does have heart issues associated with it which may be a concern for the elderly.

Anti-anxiety Medications

Anti-anxiety medications are also known as minor tranquilizers, anxiolytics and sedative-hypnotics. They are commonly prescribed for agitation in the elderly despite many studies that show they may actually add to confusion. This is because, unlike the antipsychotics, they work on the principle of sedation. At the same time, however, these medications are much more familiar to families and most non-psychiatric physicians and therefore more accepted. An as needed Ativan prescription can be commonly found in a nursing home whereas as needed Risperdal is almost unheard of. This is interesting as the literature generally supports the use of an anti-psychotic as the first line for agitation in confused people.

For the most part, these medications are in a group called benzodiazepines. Like alcohol, they are all powerful anti-anxiety agents. Consistent with the name sedative hypnotic, they are sedating and sometimes used for sleep. And, like alcohol, they are addictive and may have an associated withdrawal syndrome if stopped abruptly.

Benzodiazepines should therefore be limited to the following three uses in the elderly: for acute anxiety or panic in a relatively non-confused patient, as a second or third line sleep aid, and as an additive treatment with an anti-psychotic for extreme agitation. Let's look at some of the choices from this group.

Ativan (lorazepam) is probably the most commonly used benzodiazepine in the elderly in the US. Dosing is similar to Haldol and Risperdal, .5 to 2mg once to twice a day. Some people give it for sleep. It is commonly seen as a PRN (as needed) medication for agitation. One of the reasons it is so popular is because, like Haldol, it can be given by mouth (PO), by injection (IM), or IV. This makes it a great hospital medication. It is often given with Haldol for the management of agitation if the general hospital and on psychiatric units. Ativan can also be used for alcohol withdrawal and the acute management of seizures. It is reasonably short acting.

Xanax (alprazolam) is another popular anti anxiety medication. It is less commonly used with the elderly and often used in the younger population for panic anxiety. It cannot be given in any route other than orally but dissolves well under the tongue. Doses range from .25mg to 1mg daily in the elderly. Xanax is fairly short acting. It does not cross react with the others so a withdrawal treatment for Xanax must be done with Xanax and only Xanax.

Klonopin (clonazepam) is a longer acting benzodiazepine that is commonly used to help stabilize moods. It is usually dosed 0.5 to 3mg daily.

Valium (diazepam) is the old standard for anxiety. Doses range from 2.5mg to 10mg daily. It is not commonly used in the elderly partly because of the longer metabolism time. Valium can be given IV but is not recommended for use as an injection in the muscle.

Restoril (temazepam) is mentioned here because it is commonly given for sleep. It can only be given orally and the doses range from 15 to 30mg each night.

Halcion (triazolam) is a powerful hypnotic medication. I understand it has been banned from use in the United Kingdom due to side effect. It should never be used in the elderly.

Buspar (buspirone) is one anti-anxiety medication that is not a benzodiazepine. It was developed as an alternative to the addictive sedative hypnotics. This medication requires some time to work and is often under dosed. While generally free of side effects, Buspar is often free of being of any help as well.

Antidepressants

In terms of numbers of prescriptions, anti-depressants are likely the most widely prescribed medications in the United States. While it's true that depression is a frequent medical problem, it wasn't always the case that so many of us were taking antidepressants. Changes in the both chemistry of the medications and the way we view antidepressants have changed all that.

Like the antipsychotics, there are two groups of antidepressants: the newer and the older. The older group was very problematic. They were uncomfortable to take, often giving a variety of serious side effects. They were toxic, lethal in over doses and often sedating. In fact, it was difficult to get an older person on a therapeutic dose of an older antidepressant without making them delirious.

Starting with Wellbutrin and then Prozac in the mid eighties, the newer group has revolutionized the treatment of depression (and to some degree sensationalized it). Side effects are much less severe although still a serious consideration. Overdoses on the newer antidepressants are rarely lethal. As is true with all medications, the newer generation is much more expensive.

Old or new, antidepressants have many similarities. They work through the manipulation of neurotransmitters in the brain felt to be involved with mood. The most common of these are Serotonin and Norepinephrine. There are many choices of antidepressants, none of which has individually been shown to work better at raising mood than the others. Rather, it is the side effect profiles that are considered when deciding which might be more appropriate for a given patient. For example, a sedating antidepressant given at night might do well for a patient who is not sleeping.

Traditional antidepressants are not happy pills. They do not make you high. They are not addictive and they all take time to work. Generally, about two weeks are required before any effect on depression may be seen and this may be quite subtle. There is greater than a sixty percent response rate with antidepressants however the placebo effect (the effect seen on those placed on comparative sugar pills in studies) is about thirty percent.

While many antidepressants have sexually inhibiting side effects that are problematic for younger patients, this is less of a deal breaker in the treatment of depression in dementia. Older people with damaged brains are more sensitive to other side effects that may be seen with antidepressants such as anxiety, mania or even confusion. While not common, these side effects may require discontinuation of the medication. Antidepressants are generally tolerated in patients on a variety of other mediations and with a variety of medical problems. Let's look at the older and newer groups separately.

The Older Antidepressants

Given the modern advances, there is currently a very limited role for the older antidepressants in the treatment of depression in the elderly. In fact, many of these medications are on regulatory lists for discontinuation if identified in the elderly because of their inappropriateness. Most with dementia would not tolerate the therapeutic doses of the older antidepressants. This is because this group of medications are extremely anticholinergic, that terrible property for the elderly that we have already discussed involving dry mouth, blurred vision, constipation, urine retention and confusion. Just the stuff for grandma.....not.

We shall list several of the older antidepressants because you do still see patients from time to time who are on these medications. More commonly they are used in small doses, much less than that required for treating depression, as a sleep aide. Most of them are indeed sedating. Trazadone is in fact one of the most highly recommended sleep aides for dementia patients as it lacks the severe anticholinergic properties of the others yet is still sedating. Let's look closer at some of the older antidepressants.

Elavil (amitriptyline) is an old standard, possibly the most popular antidepressant of the sixties and seventies. Being very sedating it is still seen from time to time in low doses (25mg to 50mg) for sleep. Some doctors use it for pain in low doses as well. It is very anticholinergic.

Tofranil (imipramine) sometimes seen for sleep at 25mg to 50mg. It is very anticholinergic.

Sinequan (doxepin) also used for sleep on occasion at 25mg to 50mg. It too is very anticholinergic.

Deseryl (trazadone) is quite commonly used for sleep at 25mg to 50mg. It is well tolerated at this dose and has little anticholinergic potential. Side effects may include a drop in blood pressure upon standing and a painful pathologic erection in men known as priapism.

Other antidepressants that should never be used in dementia patients for any purpose are Nortriptyline, Desipramine and Nardil. Nardil is from a group called MAOI inhibitors. They are so dangerous that a special diet must be adhered to if taking them to avoid a high blood pressure crisis. Additionally, MAO inhibitors should never be mixed with other antidepressants.

The newer generation antidepressants.

As stated, this is a group of very effective and generally well-tolerated medications. There are many choices and side effect profiles often determine which the best to use is.

Wellbutrin (bupropion) is the oldest of the new generation. It is generally well tolerated but may be associated with anxiety at higher doses. Doses range from 75 to 300 milligrams. The extended release may be used once a day. Wellbutrin has no sexual side effects and is often used for smoking cessation in the form of Zyban.

Prozac (fluoxetine), other than penicillin, is probably the most influential medication of the twentieth century. Despite a successful campaign by some religious groups to deteriorate its value, Prozac has been a very successful medication. It does have a very long life in the blood stream (a half life of weeks) making it less desirable in the elderly because the need to get medications out of the system quickly at times. Prozac is very activating and a good choice for a severly-depressed patient who might die if not mobilized. Because of its activation, Prozac should always be given in the morning in doses of 10 to 40 milligrams. It is also indicated for bulimia and panic disorder in the US.

Zoloft (sertraline) came out in the early nineties just after Prozac. This extremely popular medication can be problematic in elderly patients sometimes causing hallucinations and diarrhea. It is not particularly activating or sedating. Doses are generally 25 to 200 milligrams. It is also indicated for Obsessive compulsive disorder in the US.

Paxil (paroxetine) is another very popular medication. This medication is often given for anxiety as well. Paxil can be somewhat sedating and is more anticholinergic than the others. It should usually be given at night. Dosage is 10 to 30 milligrams. Paxil is also indicated for Obsessive compulsive disorder and Post Traumatic Stress Disorder in the US.

Celexa (citalopram) is the European Prozac. FDA approval for use in the United States was given in the late nineties. Celexa is a favorite for the elderly because of its tolerability. Dose at 20mg to 40mg.

Lexapro (escitalopram) is essentially left handed Celexa. This medication was formulated because the right-handed form of the molecule had less therapeutic value and was the cause of many of the side effects. It is well tolerated in the elderly and is indicated for anxiety treatment in the US.

Effexor (venlafaxine) is a very popular medication that some doctor's use predominantly. It can produce anxiety and confusion in the elderly in high doses. The extended release may be used for once a day dosing. Doses range from 75 to 225 milligrams daily.

Pristiq (desvenlafaxine) is a very new antidepressant that appears to be fairly well tolerated in the elderly. Dosage is 50mg daily.

Cymbalta (duloxetine) is an antidepressant with three indications in the US that make is quite useful in the elderly: depression, anxiety and neuropathic pain. It appears to be well tolerated and is dosed as 30 to 60mg daily.

Remeron (mirtazapine) has become very popular with dementia patients. It can be given alone or with another antidepressant in severe cases. Its primary side effects, sedation and appetite stimulation, are often taken advantage of in doses of 15mg and 30mg for patients who are not eating or sleeping well. One loses these side effects at the highest dose of 45mg making this a more practical dose for younger patients. It has no sexual side effects.

Ritalin (methylphenidate) is a close relative to amphetamine. While often used for Attention Deficit Disorder in children and not officially an antidepressant, it has a use in the elderly. Given in AM doses of 5mg to 20mg, it can lift spirits and mobilize a severely depressed patient while waiting for traditional antidepressants to work. This may be life saving as some elderly depressed patients cannot survive two weeks if not mobilized. Ritalin can cause anxiety but is generally well tolerated in low dosages. Note that this medication is highly is addicting. As with all medications, the risks and benefits must be weighed by the physician, patient and family.

Mood Stabilizers

Mood stabilizing medications are commonly used for management of bipolar or manic depressive illness. They can also be useful in other conditions where mood instability occurs. Dementia is commonly associated with mood swings as well as agitation.

The classic medication in this group is Lithium. Lithium is an element that comes in a variety of salt forms such as Lithium Carbonate or Lithium Citrate which is a solution. There is also a long lasting form of lithium known as Eskalith that is a long lasting preparation. While still used in some cases of bipolar illness in younger people, Lithium has been replaced by other safer medications with less potential for toxicity and kidney damage. All the non-lithium mood stabilizers other than the antipsychotics discussed previously are also anticonvulsants and used for the treatment of seizures. Note that starting one of these medications will likely change the blood levels of other seizure medications. It is very important to monitor those levels carefully to avoid toxicity or a seizure.

Depakote (valproic acid) is used commonly as an anticonvulsant and is a common mood stabilizer in the elderly. It is generally well tolerated but can have side effects of drowsiness and falls. Other problems rarely can involve the liver and pancreas. Blood levels are often monitored to ensure attainment of therapeutic levels of the medication however these values have much less importance in the treatment of mood disorders as with management of seizures. Doses generally range from 125mg twice a day to 1000mg twice a day in the elderly.

Tegretol (carbamazepine) is an anticonvulsant as well. It too, has measurable blood levels. Tegretol is well tolerated but can have an uncommon side effect of shutting down the bone marrow production of red blood cells (aplastic anemia). For this reason monitoring of red blood cells is crucial. Dosing is at 100 to 800 milligrams twice daily.

Neurontin (gabapentin) is well tolerated with few side effects. It is less useful in my experience for the management of mood disorders however may have a dual purpose in helping with pain from diabetic neuropathy. Dosing is generally from 150 to 300 milligrams twice a day.

Lamictal (lamotrigine) is another anticonvulsant used for the stabilization of moods. Rash is a common side effect. Dosing is 25 to 100 milligrams twice daily.

Klonopin (clonazepam) is actually an antianxiety medication but does seem to have some benefit in stabilizing moods. Dosing is 0.5 to 3mg daily.

Sleep Medications

Sleep is crucial to all of us and is often disturbed in dementia. The cause of a sleep disturbance can be very complex. A paranoid psychosis, where someone is up all night suspiciously monitoring a situation is not rare but a chronic night owl's nighttime habits may be at play as well. And sometimes there is no explanation for poor sleep except that a severely confused, agitated and miserable patient is wandering about at all hours of the night. Sundowning, an increase in the afternoon and evening confusion in dementia patients, may contribute to poor sleep as well.

There are often available behavioral and environmental options that should be attempted before using medication for sleep in dementia patients. An assessment of the room environment for noise and temperature problems that cannot be articulated by the patient should always be considered. Pain should also be a consideration as well as bowel and urination issues. While some allowance for night-time wandering may be necessary in some patients, the lack of sleep at night will more often than not create daytime problems such as irritability, agitation, and a worsening of psychosis. Avoidance of daytime napping can be helpful but will often lead to caregiver fatigue unless there is considerable staff available. Sooner or later medication must be considered for any substantial sleeping problem.

An initial strategy may be to make changes with current medications. Most antipsychotics, antianxiety medications, and many antidepressants have some sedating properties. Also, there are some members of each class that are more sedating than others. Most such medication should be given at night if dosed only once a day. Prozac and Abilify are exceptions.

Similarly, if a patient is on no psychiatric medication, one may attempt to identify a problem that might be contributing to the sleeplessness such as psychosis, anxiety or depression and start a new medication from the appropriate class that will address the sleep problem as well.

With a couple exceptions, specific medications for sleep are generally drawn out of two groups - older sedating antidepressants and antianxiety medications. Of the first group, Trazadone dosed from 25mg to 100mg is widely accepted. Many patients may experience some sleepiness the next day however a worsening of confusion generally does not occur. Other older antidepressant medications such as Elavil or Sinequan are sedating but also very anticholinergic and can lead to a worsening of confusion or even delirium.

Restoril is the benzodiazepine most commonly used for sleep. It can lead to some next day sleepiness, it is potentially addicting, and like any benzodiazepine has the potential to make a patient delirious. Ativan, Xanax or even valium are used on occasion although these are second or third line choices because of problems with delirium and over sedation associated with benzodiazepines. Halcion (triazolam) is a dangerous medication and should not be used.

Newer sedatives such as Ambien (zolpidem) have been used successfully in some cases. Seroquel, an antipsychotic, is particularly useful for sleepless sundowners at doses of 25 to 100 milligrams at night. Melatonin 3mg nightly is appealing to many because it is natural and is commonly used successfully.

Pain medications

This is a subject unto itself but I will touch on it as pain may be a serious problem in patients with dementia. Older people may have a multitude of problems causing pain such as arthritis, broken bones from falls or even bedsores. Dementia patients are often unable to express their pain verbally. This makes the diagnosis and treatment of the pain in this group particularly challenging. Additionally, due to sensitivities in the elderly to medication, side effects such as stomach distress, sedation, and falls may be complicating factors. Tylenol is often considered a good place to start because of the lack of gastric erosion and ulcers.

Other options at this level include the NSAIDS (non-steroidal anti-inflammatory drugs) that include aspirin (Ecotrin), ibuprofen (Motrin or Advil), and Naprosyn (Aleve). The major problem with the NSAIDS is the potential for erosion of the gastric mucosa (lining of the stomach). One may note that many patients are on aspirin as well to help avoid blood clots in people with certain medical problems. These medications are not sedating and have little addictive potential.

Another group generally considered at the level Tylenol and the NSAIDS but which work somewhat differently is the COX2 inhibitors. COX2 is an enzyme involved in transmission of pain. These medications inhibit this enzyme thus helping to relieve one of pain. Recently, Vioxx, one of the more popular of these medications was taken off the market in the US due to evidence it may increase heart disease. Others in this group have been implicated as well although there is no evidence that they too may increase heart attacks. The most popular medication in this group in the US is Celebrex.

Most other medications are narcotic in nature. They have addiction potential, are all sedating at a high enough dosage, cause constipation, and may cause delirium. Many choices are available including some very well know products such as Vicoden, Percocet, Oxycontin, Darvocet. Morphine and methadone are also used on occasion in the elderly. The fentanyl patch (Duragesic) is a way to avoid the use of pills. It is given as 12.5 – 100 micrograms every 72 hours.

Vitamins and Natural Products

Yikes! This is another area that could take up a book or two or three. How about a thousand? That's about how many there are; many with differing opinions and angles. I do think we would agree that a multivitamin program is a good idea for all us and particularly the elderly. There are few studies that support aggressive use of vitamins or other natural products as a means of treating dementia. Certainly, vitamin B12 deficiency may mimic dementia and needs to be replaced in deficiency states. Ample vitamin b12 generally can otherwise be gotten from a normal diet. There is a thiamine (vitamin B1) deficiency associated with alcohol dementia called Wernicke syndrome that responds well to thiamine replacement.

There was one study showing that 2000mg of Vitamin E daily may prevent nursing home placement 6 months. This led to a common practice of administering vitamin E to all those with dementia. There have been several studies since that failed to support its value. Its use has most recently lost favor especially considering a potentially toxic interaction between this vitamin and Coumadin.

I hold a high bar when it comes to dementia treatment because there is no time to waste. A replicated randomized controlled double blind study in the New England Journal of Medicine in the US or the Lancet in the UK would get my attention. I know of no such study when it comes to vitamins, natural products or nutritional styles.

Chapter 18

Dementia prevention

Other than the certainty of specific genetic disorders such as Huntington's or the relatively rare "familial" form of Alzheimer's disease, genetics are way down the list of relative risk factors for the development of dementia in each of us. That is good because genes generally cannot be prevented. But there is no known prevention of Alzheimer's disease either. Fortunately, it is probably the case that atherosclerotic disease and oxidative stress play a large role in dementia by either supporting the development of Alzheimer's disease, causing vascular dementia, or both. This notion is suggested by the known risk factors for developing dementia in general. These include age, high blood pressure, high cholesterol, and diabetes. It is likely that cigarette smoking, diets high in fat and carbohydrates and alcoholism are contributors as well. Most of these conditions (except alcoholism) have been implicated in the development of atherosclerosis. Given that little is known about preventative measures for Alzheimer's disease itself, it makes sense that we should focus on caring for our blood vessels and general well-being of our brains.

Non-medication preventative activities are well known and important. Clearly a diet that is low in refined sugar and processed carbohydrates will help limit the development of diabetes. Low animal fat diets that contain high amounts of fish are well known to limit the development of fatty plaque as well. Supplements that will lower oxidative stress and thus degenerative processes include products that balance the fatty acid contents in our bodies such as fish oil and flax oil. Resveratrol, found red wine, berries and other fruits appears to be a powerful anti-oxidant as well. Vitamin D, which is actually a hormone produced in our body, has been found to require supplementation in a very high percentage of the population. This deficiency has been linked to brain health issues including dementia.

Exercise is well known to limit the development of atherosclerosis as is cessation from cigarettes. Obviously, avoiding toxic inhalants is recommended too. In my mind the jury is out when it comes to mental exercise and dementia prevention. It only makes sense that circuits might be stronger and that there might be more of them (or something like that) if we do more mental exercises. It has been shown that stroke patients are able to create new channels of brain activity over time. But one only has to realize that high IQ or high levels of mental activity do not seem to statistically prevent dementia to question this idea; however much we would like to believe it is true.

And then there is alcohol. This would not be an issue is people didn't like to drink. It doesn't help that we have a naturally occurring enzyme in our body called alcohol dehydrogenase that breaks down the ethanol and allows us to tolerate it. It almost seems as though we were meant to drink. Let's be clear, alcohol is a brain toxin. There may be some prevention of platelet aggregation and thus blood clotting at low levels and red wine does have Resveratrol but there are other sources of that. In the end, while there is some dispute about low to moderate intake, there is no doubt that higher doses cause dementia. We must each decide how to move forward with that information in mind.

Recent evidence also suggests that cholesterol-lowering drugs such as Lipitor or Zocor might be associated with prevention of dementia. Certainly this is true to the extent that these medications, also known as statins, prevent the development of atherosclerotic plaques and thus the vascular events that take their toll on brain cells. Additionally however, there seems to be something more with these medications that slows the development of the degeneration seen in

Alzheimer's dementia. These medications are currently being studied to evaluate this claim further.

Dementia prevention is an arena with a lot of buzz particularly on the internet. One needs to be careful about what is and what is not. Take for example the longtime understanding by scientists that the Amyloid protein killed the brain cells in Alzheimer dementia. This has been a central hypothesis of the disease mechanism. Well, as I understand it from a reliable scientific source, the plaques were recently experimentally removed in animal studies and it didn't prevent the disease. There is clearly much that we all have to learn.

Chapter 19

Legal issues

Involuntary commitment

From time to time there are patients who are so out of control that they cannot be willfully treated. Involuntary commitment is the ultimate place to manage this problem. Being that it is by definition, against somebodies will, one might imagine that the patient is either against the commitment or so disturbed that they are unable to understand what is happening to them. This can create very unique ethical and legal problems.

In the US, each state has their own laws regulating involuntary commitment with considerable variability between them. For example, in New York State, a Two Physician Certificate or 2PC is often used. This requires that two licensed physicians and a family member or hospital administrator agree that the patient would benefit from an involuntary hospitalization. The patient has an immediate right to a lawyer and a court hearing within one week. It is also possible for any one physician to hold a person for 48 hours if a life is in danger. As you can see in New York, the law very much supports commitment as a physician driven clinical procedure that, in the case of a 2 PC has a very broad scope.

Let's next look to the other side of the country. In Washington State the physician plays no major role in the commitment process other than making an initial referral. This referral might also be made by a nurse or social worker and must be directed to a County Designated Mental Health Professional or CDMHP. This person, not a physician, will hear the case over the telephone and assess the appropriateness of the referral. They may choose to give advice or resources over the telephone or they may chose to see the patient. They are often busy and the actual arrival for assessment may take hours to days. Meanwhile, an emergency room or skilled nursing facility has to manage a probably agitated or disturbed patient with limited legal options. Often times the CDMHP, if they see the patient will refuse commitment because the patient did not meet the specific requirements for being an immediate danger to self or others. If they do chose to commit, the patient theoretically is transferred to a hospital where they can be appropriately managed. But beds are often not available and this can be delayed for days. A court hearing will usually occur within a number of days.

Having worked extensively in both systems I can tell say that one works very well and that State has clearly dedicated resources to see that patients are treated appropriately and effectively. The other situation is very problematic and actually an embarrassment from a mental health perspective. Dementia patients are often placed far down on the food chain as they are seen as less of a risk to others.

So what does this mean for those with dementia? When they are committed, it is generally for a shorter stay for one. It is the nature of psychiatric care of dementia patients that once a treatment is formulated and implemented there can usually be some progress made soon. This is fortunate as it is truly sad to see a confused elderly person mixed in with and group of younger stronger psychotic patients.

The reality is that much of dementia care is involuntary already. Because of the confusion that dementia patients have, they may be demanding to get out of a skilled nursing facility one minute and then cooperative the next. Or they may be just kind of marginally able to understand where and why there are there all the time. Such individuals are being committed off the record so to speak by virtue of their confusion. The reality is that most patients in a nursing home have every right to walk out of there, go down to the corner bar and have a beer. Yet the doors are wired with alarms, the patients have "wander-guard" wrist bands, and some doors are actually locked.

While it is appropriate and necessary to have this security in most cases, this situation is demonstrative of the huge loop hole that exists for the elderly. Obviously it would not be cost effective or even necessary to go through a long legal process with each individual patient. It is important to remember that confused patients have rights but clearly, legal positions must be taken by someone to protect the patient and make decisions on their behalf. We have discussed the need for us all to have documentation about our specific desires relative to resuscitation and other life support care. Other decisions can be more complex.

Power of attorney

Power of attorney is a way for a person to give another person power to make decisions of their behalf should they become incapacitated by a medical condition or die. It may be restricted to money or social matters only or be broadened to include medical decisions.

In the US, rules vary from state to state relative to the issue of Power of Attorney.
An interesting aspect of power of attorney is that it often requires that a person be competent to make the decision to give someone power of attorney. Once a person is no longer able to make his or her own choices they can no longer assign as power of attorney. A guardianship should then be applied for at which point competency becomes an issue.

Competency

Competency is a legal term. It is a formal declaration that only a judge can give. Generally the process of determining competency occurs in a competency hearing where various individuals such as the family, lawyers and physicians will give their opinions about a person's capacity to make decisions. Often a psychiatrist will be asked to examine the patient and give their opinion as well.

Guardianship

A guardianship generally allows for the same control as a power of attorney. The main difference is that it has been determined by a court process. It is usually full in scope as allows allowing for the same power that one has with both medical and financial power of attorney. In certain cases a lawyer may accept the role of guardian ad litem. This is a temporary role where the patient is assessed for guardianship needs. In such cases a family may not be available to assume guardianship and potential candidates such as family friends or guardianship services are identified and evaluated to assume the duty. The role of the guardian often requires regular documentation and presentation of records to insure the continued quality involvement on the part of the guardian.

Lightning Source UK Ltd.
Milton Keynes UK
UKOW051005050212

186703UK00001B/5/P